Global Epidemics,
Local Implications

Global Epidemics, Local Implications

African Immigrants and the Ebola Crisis in Dallas

Kevin J. A. Thomas

Johns Hopkins University Press   Baltimore

© 2019 Johns Hopkins University Press
All rights reserved. Published 2019
Printed in the United States of America on acid-free paper
9 8 7 6 5 4 3 2 1

Johns Hopkins University Press
2715 North Charles Street
Baltimore, Maryland 21218-4363
www.press.jhu.edu

Library of Congress Cataloging-in-Publication Data

Names: Thomas, Kevin J. A., author.
Title: Global epidemics, local implications : African immigrants and
    the Ebola crisis in Dallas / Kevin J. A. Thomas.
Description: Baltimore : Johns Hopkins University Press, 2019. |
    Includes bibliographical references and index.
Identifiers: LCCN 2019007923 | ISBN 9781421432991 (hardcover : alk.
    paper) | ISBN 1421432994 (hardcover : alk. paper) | ISBN
    9781421433004 (electronic) | ISBN 1421433001 (electronic)
Subjects: | MESH: Hemorrhagic Fever, Ebola—ethnology | Hemor-
    rhagic Fever, Ebola—transmission | African Americans | Disease
    Outbreaks | Emigrants and Immigrants | Sociological Factors |
    Africa, Western—ethnology | Texas—epidemiology
Classification: LCC RC140.5 | NLM WC 534 | DDC 616.9/18—dc23
LC record available at https://lccn.loc.gov/2019007923

A catalog record for this book is available from the British Library.

*Special discounts are available for bulk purchases of this book. For
more information, please contact Special Sales at 410-516-6936 or
specialsales@press.jhu.edu.*

Johns Hopkins University Press uses environmentally friendly book
materials, including recycled text paper that is composed of at least
30 percent post-consumer waste, whenever possible.

Contents

Acknowledgments

Writing a book on one of the most significant public health emergencies in recent years requires so many things to go right. As such, I am grateful to God for providing me with the resources and opportunities that were needed to make this work possible. When I learned about the spread of Ebola during the early stages of the epidemic, my first reaction was of concern for the lives of those living in the affected communities. However, following the localized outbreak in Dallas, it became increasingly difficult for me to avoid viewing the crisis from the perspective of my various research interests. As a scholar whose work focuses on race, ethnicity, and migration, I had several questions about the specific ways in which communities were reacting to the epidemic. One of these was the question of how many African immigrants in Dallas were responding to the disruptions caused by Ebola in the two transatlantic contexts to which they were connected. In my search for answers, I decided to go to Dallas to conduct research to examine how this response unfolded.

Two sources of funding obtained from the Pennsylvania State University were used to support my research in the city. The African Research Center provided me with generous funds through its faculty grants program, which supports research that examines the lives of Africans across the diaspora. These funds were used to cover the expenses associated with the first phase of my research in Dallas in the early summer of 2016. Later that summer, I conducted the second phase of my research in the city, with additional funds provided by the African Studies program.

When I first arrived in Dallas, I knew no one in the city, although I had the contact information of a few community leaders I had called to inform about my project. In the subsequent weeks, however, my work was greatly advanced by the generosity of members of the African immigrant community. By the time I left, they had taken me to their churches, invited me into their homes, and allowed me to meet with their leaders. While conducting my research, I was also invited to eat various African delicacies, such as foofoo and egusi soup, puff-puffs, and jollof rice. Indeed, the hospitality I received was remarkable. I truly appreciate the willingness of Africans in Dallas to welcome me into their lives.

Although I cannot name all the people who offered their assistance to me while I was in Dallas, there are several who deserve special mention. Patrick Jackson, the honorary consul of Sierra Leone in Dallas, was instrumental in getting me information on the various West African immigrant associations found in the city. Nathan Kortu and Dr. Emanuel Botchway helped to ease my entry into the Liberian immigrant community and introduced me to key leaders who participated in their larger response to the epidemic. Dr. Sanmi Akinmulero, president and CEO of the African Chamber of Commerce in the Dallas–Fort Worth area, was kind enough to allow me to attend weekly meetings of his organization. These meetings provided me with an opportunity to meet with the owners of various African small-scale businesses in Dallas. Several individuals also helped to set up interviews, introduce me to key informants, and provide suggestions of leaders I should consider interviewing. The most notable of these facilitators were Waltona Cummings, Stanley Gaye, David Kassebeh, Juma Kayembe, and Clavenda Pratt.

I also benefited from complimentary assistance provided by various nonimmigrant institutions in Dallas. These include the Africa Program at the University of Texas, Arlington; Catholic Charities of Dallas; the Dallas Public Library; the International Rescue Committee; Vickery Meadow Youth Development Foundation; and Wilshire Baptist Church. As a result of their assistance, I was able to identify official documents, better understand the work of humanitarian organizations serving the African community in the city, and gain critical insight into the city's experience during the 2014 Ebola outbreak.

Various scholars at Pennsylvania State University and Southern Methodist University played a role in helping me develop my ideas during various stages of the project. At Pennsylvania State University, they include my colleagues in the African Studies program, the Department of Sociology and Criminology, and the Population Research Institute's Immigration

Working Group. As I tried to make sense of the information I collected during my research, I received first-class assistance from Dr. Christopher Inkpen, then a doctoral student in the Department of Sociology and Criminology. Several scholars at Southern Methodist University in Dallas willingly shared their expertise on the African immigrant population in the city. These individuals include Dr. Jill Kelly of the Department of History and Dr. Caroline Brettell and Dr. Carolyn Smith-Morris of the Department of Anthropology. I am further grateful to Dr. Carolyn Smith-Morris for reading one of my earliest chapters and subsequently providing her feedback.

My family deserves special mention for the support they provided as I worked to make this book a reality. My wife, Tina, was always willing to listen to my ideas, read drafts of the manuscript, and ask critical questions I needed to answer to remind me to convey my ideas in terms accessible to a nontechnical audience. My daughters, Abigail and Lydia, had words of encouragement that helped to keep me focused on what I was trying to accomplish. Additionally, my elderly parents' desire to read this book when it is published inspired me in ways that words cannot fully express.

Finally, I would like to thank Robin Coleman and the staff of Johns Hopkins University Press for shepherding me through the process of publishing this book. Their assistance was nothing but stellar and was instrumental in helping me complete this book on the experiences of African immigrants in Dallas during the recent Ebola epidemic.

Global Epidemics,
Local Implications

1 International Migration, Ebola, and Responses to Global Epidemics

L eft behind from recent economic progress in Guinea, Meliandou is far removed from the bright lights of Conakry, the country's capital city. Most of its residents are poor rural farmers, and unpaved roads carefully wind their way up toward the village's location on a hill. There is only one working well serving the village, and like many farming communities in Guinea, Meliandou lacks good schools, a modern hospital, and the most basic social services (Faul 2014). Yet none of this matters to children in the village when it is time to get together to play. With few recreational options available, they most frequently play around the area near a cola tree. For as long as anyone can remember, though, the tree has been home to dozens of bats, but this is not unusual in the forest region of Nzérékoré. Toward the end of December 2013, Emile Ouamouno, a two-year-old boy who lived about fifty meters from the tree, died after a short illness. His cause of death was unknown, but it set off a chain of events that had far-reaching consequences in Guinea and beyond.

Within a month of his death, Emile's three-year-old sister, mother, and grandmother died of a hemorrhagic fever. Shortly thereafter, several extended family members who attended the funerals of the deceased became ill and died. Two healthcare workers who had taken care of the sick soon became infected by a mysterious disease. They also died after short illnesses. Unknown to Meliandou's residents, the disease had started to spread beyond the borders of the village. Gbandou and Dawa were nearby villages from which people had traveled to Meliandou to attend the funeral of Emile's grandmother. A few weeks after they returned home, reports emerged that individuals from those villages had been afflicted with an unknown infection and died relatively quickly after. Back in Meliandou, the village midwife who provided care for Emile's family became sick and needed someone to care for her, and a relative from another village, Dandou Pombo, came by to do just that. After she returned, there were reports from her village of a new mysterious illness that caused the deaths of six people; they all died relatively quickly after becoming infected (Gholipour 2014).

By early January 2014, the growing number of deaths from the mysterious disease had become alarming. Meliandou residents were troubled by what was occurring, but there was very little they could do. Their small health post lacked the resources needed to investigate the causes of the increasing spate of deaths. Running out of options, they informed district officials about the strange sequence of fatal events that were preceded by severe cases of diarrhea. After conducting their own investigations, these officials concluded that there was no reason to be alarmed, since the symptoms of the deceased were quite similar to those of cholera. Consequently, no extra precaution was taken; there was no need to overreact because cholera was common in the region (World Health Organization [WHO] 2015c).

With no action taken to identify the true cause of the infections, the budding epidemic continued to spread. A healthcare worker who provided care for infected persons in the villages of Gbandou and Dawa became ill and subsequently traveled to the nearby town of Macenta. The town was the closest location with a modern hospital, and it was about fifty-five miles from the town of Gueckedou, where the nongovernmental organization Médecins Sans Frontières (MSF) was conducting a malaria project. By the start of March 2014, hospitals in both Macenta and Gueckedou were receiving large numbers of patients with an unknown infection. They all had a consistent set of symptoms: acute cases of diarrhea, high fevers, and frequent vomiting followed by death shortly after becoming infected. Three of these deaths occurred at the Gueckedou hospital, along with an unspecified number of deaths among patients and workers at the hospital in Macenta (Baize et al. 2014).

Employees in both hospitals were so concerned about the deaths that they notified officials at the Guinean Ministry of Health and MSF. During its long history of working on humanitarian emergencies, MSF had provided care to victims of Ebola during previous outbreaks in Africa. Yet, none of these outbreaks had occurred in Guinea, and all of them were contained before reaching large population centers. With assistance from WHO, MSF and the Guinean government conducted a more systematic investigation into the cause of the outbreak toward the end of March. By this time, similar cases were emerging in other areas of Guinea, including in four subdistricts in the country, as well as in Conakry, the capital city. Blood samples taken from infected patients were sent to laboratories in Lyon, France, and Hamburg, Germany, for testing (Baize et al. 2014; WHO 2015c). The first set of definitive results was received from the Institut Pasteur in Lyon, and it confirmed the cause of the mysterious illness. It was Ebola, and the specific causative agent of the virus was the Zaire species. This was the most lethal strand of Ebola known to humankind (WHO 2015c).

Considered to be among the most lethal of infectious diseases, Ebola is a zoonotic disease transmitted to humans after they come into contact with infected birds and animals (Pourrut et al. 2005). It was first discovered in 1976 after a near-simultaneous outbreak of the disease in Sudan and in what was then eastern Zaire. The disease was named after the Ebola River, located near Yambuku, and until 2013, previous epidemics had mostly occurred in rural communities in Central and Eastern Africa (Pourrut et al. 2005). On average, between 30 and 90 percent of persons affected by the virus die within twenty-one days of being infected. Since 1976, however, more than twenty species of Ebola have been identified in large-scale epidemics across Africa (Li and Chen 2014). Over this period, the highest number of deaths observed in a single epidemic was 280 (Brantly, Brantly, and Thomas 2015).

Bats are the most common nonhuman hosts of the disease, and experts believe that the 2014 West African Ebola epidemic started after the virus was transmitted to Emile Ouamouno while playing near the cola tree in Meliandou (Garrett 2015). After its transmission to humans, Ebola is transmitted between persons by direct contact with the bodily fluids of other infected persons. Its spread is accelerated because the virus is difficult to detect in the early stages of an infection. Initial identification of the virus is further complicated because many of its symptoms, including fever, vomiting, and severe diarrhea, are also symptoms of other tropical diseases such as Lassa fever, malaria, and cholera (Baize at al. 2014). For these reasons, misdiagnoses of Ebola patients are quite common, and this delays efforts to curb the spread of the virus before it becomes an epidemic.

While Ebola was confirmed as the cause of the mysterious illness in Guinea in March 2014, it was not until August 2014 that WHO declared the outbreak to be an international health emergency (Davis 2014). By this time, the virus had reached multiple countries, and the ensuing epidemic had generated significant fears about the risk of transmission from infected persons. These fears were as real in Africa as they were in America, especially after it became clear that population mobility was the major mechanism through which the virus was spread across countries.

Focusing on the global dimensions of the West African Ebola epidemic, this book pays particular attention to the significance of international migration for understanding community responses to the disease. In the United States, no immigrant group was affected by the epidemic as much as Africans in the Dallas–Fort Worth area. This area is home to many immigrants from the West African countries that were at the epicenter of the epidemic. More importantly, it was the area where the first Ebola death in US history was recorded. This book examines the experiences of African immigrants during the crisis in Dallas to better understand how epidemics in one part of the world can affect the lives of people in another. It makes no claim that the crisis in the city is representative of other epidemics linked to immigrant communities. Instead, it uses these events as part of an explanatory case study (Yin 2013) to highlight the implications of global connections for the diverse community responses observed in Dallas.

This book further illuminates the implications of spatial interconnections between places during epidemics, and it demonstrates the salience of global migration processes for understanding these implications. These processes are examined from several perspectives. Many accounts of the role of migration during epidemics focus on its obvious influence on increasing the size of populations exposed to infection. However, as this book details, migration processes are also associated with societal responses to immigrant communities during global epidemics. In most cases, these responses are negative, and previous accounts present immigrants as passive victims of these negative responses. I argue that while this perspective on the social implications of epidemics is important, it is nevertheless limiting. It ignores the fact that immigrants play an active role in these responses, and that they can take deliberate actions to shape the narrative on the consequences of diseases within their communities.

The Unfolding of an International Crisis

By the time WHO acknowledged that the crisis in Guinea had become an outbreak of Ebola, a critical mass of infected people was unknowingly transmitting the virus across international boundaries. It was during these early stages that the first reports emerged that patients with Ebola-like symptoms were being observed in neighboring countries. The first evidence confirming the international spread of the virus came at the end of March 2014, when two Ebola cases were identified in Liberia (Davis 2014). Two months later, the first case of Ebola was confirmed in Sierra Leone. Both Liberia and Sierra Leone share international borders with Guinea. As such, the early trend of the international transmission of the virus suggested that the next country in which cases would be found would most likely share a border with one of these countries.

Surprisingly, the next country to which the epidemic spread lacked a common border with Liberia and Sierra Leone. In July 2014, the first case of Ebola in Nigeria was confirmed after Patrick Sawyer arrived in the country's commercial capital, Lagos, on a flight from Monrovia, Liberia. Sawyer was a dual citizen of Liberia and the United States, as well as an employee of the Liberian steel company ArcelorMittal. Before leaving for Nigeria, he had provided care for his sister, who died after a short illness, during which she showed many of the symptoms of Ebola. Reports suggest that he traveled out of the country because he knew he was infected and desired to seek treatment in a country with more advanced healthcare facilities.* Sawyer left for Nigeria, without the approval of his employer, about two weeks after becoming infected (Ibekwe 2014b). By then, he had started to experience symptoms of the disease. Security cameras at the airport in Monrovia showed him deliberately attempting to avoid contact with other passengers before boarding his flight (Ibekwe 2014a). After arriving in Lagos, he collapsed and was rushed to the First Consultants Hospital,

---

* The wife of Patrick Sawyer maintained that he traveled to Nigeria because he was searching for a country with a better healthcare system, since he did not trust the Liberian healthcare system (Ibekwe 2014b).

where he later died. Subsequent tests confirmed that he had contracted Ebola, but by then the virus had been transmitted to several hospital personnel. Within a few weeks of his death, at least twenty people infected with Ebola were identified in Nigeria. All of them were traced to Sawyer, and six of these cases resulted in fatalities (Igonoh 2015).

The speed with which the Ebola virus spread across West Africa was alarming. This was the first time the epidemic had crossed so many international borders in Africa, and no one knew when it would end. Ebola cases in Lagos were of particular concern. With more than twelve million residents, it is the largest city in Africa, and it has advanced transportation links that connect it to global cities. As the first Ebola case in Lagos demonstrated, modern systems of transportation can allow a virus to spread from one country to a more distant location, skipping the nearest neighboring countries in the process. This combination of a deadly virus, air travel, and international population mobility had serious implications for the global spread of Ebola.

In order to counter the growing threat of the virus, several countries adopted travel bans, restricting the entry of nationals from countries affected by the crisis. One of the first countries to impose such restrictions was Liberia, because its government was concerned about the consequences of the immigration of infected persons from Guinea and Sierra Leone. Beyond Liberia, however, there was considerable variation in the types of travel restrictions adopted by countries across the globe. They ranged from the closure of borders and the suspension of visa application processes to enhanced health screenings of passengers arriving from Ebola-affected countries (Poletto et al. 2014). Altogether, thirty-three countries had imposed one or more such restrictions by November 2014, and the majority of them were in Africa (Thompson and Torre 2014). Besides the effects of these restrictions, international travel was negatively affected after several major airlines suspended their operations in Guinea, Liberia, and Sierra Leone. British Airways and Air France temporarily suspended their services to Freetown and Monrovia,* while Kenya Airways suspended flights to both cities out of concern that the scale of the outbreak was vastly un-

---

* More than seven hundred Air France workers signed a petition asking their employer to suspend travel to Ebola-affected countries in Africa (Plautz 2014).

derestimated (Anderson 2014). In general, estimates indicate that 216 of 519 monthly scheduled flights to Guinea, Liberia, and Sierra Leone were canceled around the peak of the epidemic (Anderson 2014).

Humanitarian aid agencies were opposed to these restrictions, partly due to their implications for the success of aid operations. Flight cancellations interfered with the mobility of aid workers and the delivery of supplies to affected countries. At the same time, the very premise of the restrictions was unsubstantiated. Studies on their potential effect on curbing the spread of the epidemic suggested that they were ineffective and were only likely to delay the international spread of the virus by a few weeks (Poletto et al. 2014).

Notwithstanding the growing fears about the potential spread of the virus, all deaths to infected persons had occurred in countries close to the source of the epidemic in West Africa. As it spread to other countries beyond Nigeria, however, the epidemic's connection to international migration became more evident. In Mali, which lies across the northern border of Guinea, the first Ebola case was that of a two-year-old girl whose family returned to the country after traveling to neighboring Guinea. The girl's father, who was also from Mali, worked as a healthcare provider in Guinea. He had provided care for a Guinean farmer who later died from undiagnosed causes, but he became sick himself and died a few days after showing symptoms of the virus (WHO 2014b). A relative from Kayes, in Mali, traveled to Guinea to offer her condolences to the family of the deceased. She returned to Mali with the young child, not knowing that by then the child was also infected with the virus (WHO 2014b). Following their return, the virus spread to eight people and resulted in a total of six deaths.

The Ebola virus spread to Senegal under similar circumstances. A student from Guinea traveled to neighboring Senegal to visit his relatives in Dakar, the capital city. Unbeknownst to him, he had already been infected with the virus before leaving for Senegal. During his visit, he started to experience symptoms including vomiting, fever, and diarrhea, all of which are also associated with malaria. However, because the epidemic was spreading in Guinea, tests were conducted at the Institut Pasteur in Dakar to more accurately diagnose the cause of his illness. These tests confirmed that he had been infected with Ebola. Fortunately, this was the only case of the virus observed in the country (WHO 2014a).

For the first six months of the epidemic, few people would have assumed that Western countries would be the next places that Ebola patients would arrive. While Patrick Sawyer was also a US citizen at the time of his death in Nigeria, the country was just too far away for him to be perceived as a threat to the American public. In late July 2014, however, Kent Brantly, an American doctor, was diagnosed with the disease in Liberia, and this significantly increased coverage of the epidemic by the US media. As a missionary working in Liberia, Brantly was inadvertently infected with the virus while working at the Eternal Love Winning Africa (ELWA) hospital in Monrovia. To make things worse, another American, Nancy Writebol, who worked as a nurse at the same hospital, became infected with the virus a few days later. They were both part of a small staff of workers at this hospital, which was one of the leading providers of health services to Liberians during the epidemic. Most locals saw the hospital as a place where they could receive care that was both reliable and accessible. Consequently, doctors and nurses at the hospital saw a higher caseload of Ebola patients than other hospitals in Liberia.

Besides the fact that Brantly and Writebol are Americans, their infection with the virus was significant for other reasons. First, they were the first Ebola patients flown from West Africa to the United States to receive advanced medical treatment. They left Liberia in an aircraft specially designed to monitor their health and reduce transmission of the virus to others. After Dr. Brantly arrived at the Emory University Hospital in Atlanta, Georgia, he became the first American to live with the disease on US soil. Second, both individuals were the first people known to receive ZMapp, an experimental treatment for Ebola. This treatment provided an unprecedented level of survival to Ebola patients and helped Brantly and Writebol live. However, the treatment was in short supply, and it was also inaccessible to ordinary West Africans who had also been infected with the virus.

Increases in media coverage of the arrival of the two healthcare workers in Atlanta were accompanied by a notable shift in the narrative associated with the epidemic. The previous narrative, linked with a tacit disconnection from a disease in exotic lands, was replaced with one of fear. A deadly disease was now present in the United States, and no one knew what to expect. Critics maintained that the decision to bring the health workers to the United States would have tragic consequences, because the virus had a high rate of transmission from person to person (Brantly, Brantly, and Thomas 2015). Despite assurances that the US healthcare system was able to provide appropriate care for infected persons, there was an increasing perception that it would have been better to treat these infected individuals in Liberia than to risk the spread of the virus in the United States (Brantly, Brantly, and Thomas 2015). This narrative of fear had several consequences. Brantly's wife and children were stigmatized as carriers of the disease despite the fact that they left Liberia about a week before Brantly became infected (Brantly, Brantly, and Thomas 2015). Writebol was also stigmatized even after she had recovered from the disease. After her discharge from the hospital, she was uninvited from a number of events and encountered people who refused to shake her hand (Elgot 2014).

This narrative of fear was also preemptive of the social response to the impending crisis in Dallas. It foreshadowed the way in which the American public would react to the possibility that people perceived to embody a transmissible infection from Africa were living within their communities. In addition, it preempted the dynamics of a system of reactions characterized by a triumph of fear over facts and the imagined over what was real. Furthermore, it was a premonition of how subjective criteria were to be used to change the public discourse on the threat posed by immigrant communities.

Outside the United States, the perceived threat of the spread of Ebola to other Western countries increased, as did the link between Ebola infection and international population mobility. Individuals with infections traced to the West African epidemic arrived in Europe under circumstances reflecting the unique ways in which Ebola patients from high-income countries were being transported. As was the case with Brantly and Writebol, these individuals had contracted the virus while in Africa but had been flown home using sophisticated transportation arrangements to receive more advanced medical treatment. For example, William Pooley, a British volunteer nurse, was evacuated to the United Kingdom to receive medical treatment after he became infected while working with Ebola patients in Sierra Leone (Shuchman 2014). Furthermore, Miguel Pajares, a Spanish priest living in Liberia, was brought to Spain to receive treatment after becoming infected with the virus (Farmer 2014). As in the cases of Brantly and Writebol, international migration had brought these Westerners to West Africa, where they were exposed to the virus. However, they had returned home under circumstances that significantly reduced the risk of transmitting the virus to the public.

The observed patterns of the international transmission of Ebola during the early stages of the West African epidemic underscored two presumptions about a possible future course of the epidemic. First, international migration was expected to play a more significant role in the spread of the disease in West Africa, as a result of the region's porous international borders. Indeed, after the start of the epidemic in Meliandou, Guinea, four of the six West African countries to which the virus had spread shared a border with the country. Second, at least in terms of voluntary international migration, North American countries were expected to be among the least likely to be affected by the epidemic. None of the affected countries in Africa had a direct air-transportation connection to North American cities, and besides, the chances of large-scale medical evacuations of infected Africans to the United States were all but nonexistent.

The Ebola Crisis in Dallas

Two months after Brantly and Writebol returned to the United States, a Liberian national by the name of Thomas Duncan became the first person to be diagnosed with Ebola in the United States. This diagnosis came less than two weeks after he arrived in Dallas to visit his fiancée and son. Because the symptoms of Ebola are only observed after twenty-one days of an infection, he successfully passed through all the health-screening protocols used to prevent infected persons from boarding flights at the airport in Monrovia. Ten days after arriving in Dallas, however, he was diagnosed with Ebola, after experiencing symptoms of the disease.

News of Duncan's diagnosis created a new sense of fear while raising a number of questions that remained unanswered. How did an Ebola-infected person arrive in the United States from Africa without being detected? Would this diagnosis start a chain of transmission that could result in widespread deaths among Americans? Furthermore, were there other Africans living in Dallas who could potentially transmit the virus within the city? For Dallas residents, it was particularly concerning that during his short stay in the city, Duncan had lived in an immigrant neighborhood with West African residents from other countries affected by the epidemic. Besides, Duncan had gone to public places and interacted with others in his community, raising the possibility that a silent killer was rapidly spreading throughout the city. When he died on October 8, 2014, he became the first person to die of Ebola in the United States. However, the public's concerns were confirmed when it was revealed that the virus had infected two nurses at the Texas Health Presbyterian Hospital, where Duncan had been admitted.

Duncan's diagnosis provided a new basis for expanding the narrative of fear that had previously characterized the public discourse on Ebola. It led to a loss of public trust in healthcare professionals, who had repeatedly assured Americans that an Ebola outbreak in the United States was unlikely. Additionally, it raised questions about whether the US healthcare system was prepared to handle the disease. Subsequent evidence revealed that Duncan's symptoms had been repeatedly misdiagnosed during his initial visits to the hospital, and no red flags were raised when he reportedly informed hospital staff on multiple occasions that he had recently arrived from Liberia.

It is important to distinguish the ways in which Duncan's experiences were different from those of Brantly and Writebol. Compared to the latter, who are Americans, Duncan was an African whose arrival in Dallas occurred against the backdrop of recent increases in African immigration to the United States. Socioeconomically, he was also disadvantaged—he lived in one of the poorest neighborhoods in the city. Based on this association with contexts of poverty, it was easier to stigmatize Duncan than it was to stigmatize middle-class professionals such as Brantly and Writebol. Further accentuating the difference between the two sets of cases was Duncan's racial identity. Unlike these two White Americans, Duncan was Black. This difference does not imply that race was the overriding determinant of Duncan's experiences in Dallas. Instead, it suggests that we cannot ignore the fact that his experience occurred in a US healthcare system in which race has been found to be an important marker of disparity in the quality of care received by patients (Schneider et al. 2002; Williams and Wyatt 2015).

Duncan's death was emblematic of more than just the failures of the US healthcare system. It symbolized the negative effects of globalization while activating Americans' fears of the unknown. After all, he was from a country in Africa that few people had heard of, and he had successfully traveled to the United States with a mysterious disease for which there was no cure. The closest objects representing this new threat to the public were people who looked like Duncan. Accordingly, his death was followed by a widespread backlash against African immigrants living in the Dallas area.

To many people, these immigrants represented an existential threat to American life. As a result, they were ostracized, mocked, and stereotyped as carriers of the deadly disease (Brown and Constable 2014; Fuller 2015; Smith-Morris 2017). The backlash spread beyond immigrants from Liberia to other African immigrants. It was felt by immigrants from countries such as South Africa and Rwanda, because it was difficult to differentiate Liberians from other African immigrants (Terkel 2014). In some communities, the hostility against Africans was so intense that hotlines were created to report incidents of harassment (Terkel 2014). Additionally, the US Department of Justice stepped up its efforts to protect the rights of African immigrants by issuing guidelines for federal workers to guard against the possibility of discrimination against individuals perceived to be infected with the virus (Delaney 2014).

While the backlash against African immigrants was observed in other parts of the United States, the most extensive displays of anti-African sentiment were observed in Dallas. The new crisis underscored the consequences of the city's increased connectivity with other cities across the globe. In a span of eight months, a disease outbreak that started in a poor rural village in Guinea had reached a major city in one of the world's most developed nations. Only a few studies have examined how such connections across global space shape the ways in which societies respond to epidemics. Moreover, we know very little about how diaspora communities abroad respond to global epidemics that start in their origin communities. These gaps in the literature are significant and warrant new ways of understanding the social implications of infectious disease epidemics. Part of this process involves recognizing the complex nature of the relationship between international migration and the outbreak of disease.

As this book demonstrates, international migration is significant not only for understanding how epidemics are transmitted across international boundaries but also for recognizing the multidimensional responses to epidemics observed in migrant destination societies. This dual approach to grasping the social dynamics of epidemics is largely missing from accounts of previous health crises. To better understand these implications, it is important to examine what membership in transnational communities implies for the ways in which African immigrants navigated the diverse risks associated with living in Ebola contexts during their visits to West Africa. At the same time, because many immigrants continued to maintain social connections with origin communities at the center of the epidemic, their vicarious experiences with the trauma and fear experienced in these places must also be recognized. This dual approach thus requires a careful analysis of how immigrants can still be exposed to the fatal consequences of a disease outbreak in their countries of origin. Yet, it also demands an examination of how epidemics shape social relationships, public interactions, and the deployment of resources in immigrant communities abroad. Furthermore, it requires an investigation of how symbols of immigrant identity were utilized in the construction of stigmas that resulted in their exclusion from the everyday interactions that occur in their host societies.

Race was an inherent characteristic of immigrant identity closely linked to public reactions to the Ebola crisis in Dallas. Consequently, the implications of the Ebola epidemic across international space cannot be fully understood without an analysis of how racial identity, along with characteristics such as nativity status and socioeconomic disadvantage, shapes the impacts of the outbreak on diaspora communities. It is important to examine, for example, how racial stereotypes were used in the construction of stigma targeting Africans in Dallas. Similarly, the question of whether minority status provided a basis for developing partnerships with US minority groups who were exploited when responding to the crisis also needs to be addressed.

Migration, Infectious Diseases, and the Connection between Places

Concerns about the relationship between migration and the spread of Ebola partly reflect the historical recognition of the role of migration processes in the spread of disease. As far back as 430 BC, for example, international migration was considered a major determinant of the start of an epidemic in ancient Greece. Close to one hundred thousand people died during the plague of Athens, which is suspected to have originated in Ethiopia, after which it spread to Egypt and Libya before reaching the city (Salway and Dell 1955). While there is very little evidence empirically validating this suspicion, a clear connection between international migration and the spread of disease was observed in subsequent epidemics. In the Middle East in the 1330s, for example, the bubonic plague was traced to the migration of people from its source in central Asia, through China and India (Panagiotakopulu 2004). Closer to the United States, the smallpox epidemic in Hispaniola in 1518 was traced to the arrival of African slaves who worked in the island's silver mines. The ensuing epidemic killed more than half of the Indian population of the island before it spread to Cuba, Mexico, and Central America (Kohn 2007; McNeill 1998). Similar patterns continued to be observed at the turn of the twentieth century, when population movements were associated with the spread of tuberculosis in Southern Africa. Before the early 1900s, the disease was very rare in the region. However, after the arrival of miners from European countries where the disease was endemic, tuberculosis was transmitted to South Africa during an epidemic first observed among local miners (Rees et al. 2010).

As globalization increases, concerns about the role of migration in the spread of disease have taken on a new level of significance. International migration to the West has increased, while at the same time new health conditions are emerging in many migrant-sending countries. It is under these circumstances that the growth in US immigrant trends has occurred. This growth has been accompanied by notable shifts in the major sources of immigrants. Until the middle of the twentieth century, most immigrants to the United States emigrated from Europe, while more recent immigrants have come from countries in Asia, Latin America, and Africa. For the most part, the increase in emigration from these countries has occurred at a time when many of them have experienced weakening institutional support for their healthcare sectors and declines in the provision of primary healthcare services (Gushulak and MacPherson 2004).

Immigrant destinations in the West are thus among the most common contexts in which a new relationship between migration and disease is being observed, as newly arriving immigrants contribute to transformations in the local epidemiology of disease. Increases in hospitalizations for diseases such as malaria and viral hepatitis have been observed in Switzerland, and these increases have been linked to previous residence in Africa (Fenner et al. 2007). In the United States, Canada, and Spain, recent immigration trends have been linked to the emergence of new diseases such as Chagas disease. Although the disease is endemic in the Southern Hemisphere, it is believed to have spread to Europe and North America as a result of increasing emigration from South American countries due to political instability and declining living standards (Schmunis 2007). Compared to infectious diseases such as Ebola, however, Chagas is not easily spread by mere contact with infected persons. Instead, most cases of human-to-human transmission of the disease have occurred during blood and organ donations from infected persons (Schmunis 2007).

Contemporary patterns of globalization are also linked to increases in the speed with which diseases are transmitted between countries as well as an expansion of the spatial boundaries within which epidemics occur. In the 2003 severe acute respiratory syndrome (SARS) epidemic, the first case of the virus was observed in Guangdong, China, from which it was transmitted to thirty countries, including Canada, Singapore, and the United States (Centers for Disease Control and Prevention [CDC] 2003; Varia et al. 2003). Similar patterns were observed during the Middle East respiratory syndrome coronavirus (MERS-CoV) epidemic of 2012, which was less extensive in scale. In this case, the virus spread to nine countries after the first case was observed in Saudi Arabia (Wickramage et al. 2013). Such extensive patterns of the international diffusion of disease played a central role in increasing global fears about the spread of the Zika virus in 2015. Originally found in the Zika Forest in Uganda in 1947, the most recent outbreak originated in Brazil, after which the virus was transmitted to more than ten countries (Lowes 2016; Petersen et al. 2016).

At the most basic level, these viruses spread when individuals infected in one region migrate with the disease to another. For several reasons, however, the relationship between migration and the disease can be much more complicated. One reason is that many migration movements involve the circulation of people between places. When these movements occur across international borders, they are typically referred to as transnational movements. These patterns of migration introduce additional challenges to our understanding of the dynamics of the spread of disease. In part, this is because transnational migrants maintain social and economic ties in both origin and destination countries, and maintaining these ties can contribute to repeated cycles of infection and transmission across space. After tuberculosis was introduced in South Africa by European miners in the early 1900s, for example, the transmission of the disease to African miners resulted in the spread of the disease to other parts of the region due to the circulation of labor between communities (Rees et al. 2010).

Transnational migration movements were part of the reason why the early spread of Ebola during the West African epidemic was so concerning. The outbreak started in the tri-border region connecting Guinea, Liberia, and Sierra Leone (Koch 2016). However, like many borders in Africa, these borders are artificial boundaries that were imposed during the colonial period and resulted in the artificial separation of people from the same ethnic groups (Ross 2014). Most locals living in African border communities are frequently involved in circular migration movements as they travel to and from neighboring countries to visit nearby relatives. During the West African Ebola epidemic, for example, the index case traced to Meliandou occurred among a primarily Kissi-speaking group in Guinea who frequently traveled across the country's borders to visit relatives in Sierra Leone and Liberia (Koch 2016). After the virus was transmitted across these borders, internal migration within these countries resulted in its subsequent spread to large urban areas with international airports connecting travelers to destinations in other countries. By the end of the Ebola epidemic, the virus had spread to seven countries on three continents. Indeed, this was the largest number of countries ever affected during a single Ebola epidemic since the virus was discovered in the 1970s.

More generally, however, the consequential nature of migration for the spread of Ebola was somewhat apparent from evidence on the diffusion of the virus in previous epidemics. In some cases, this was seen in the mass migration of the disease vectors themselves. Before the Kikwit Ebola outbreak in the Democratic Republic of Congo (DRC) in 1995, local populations reported observing the arrival of hundreds of bats that settled among fruit trees located on an abandoned plantation in the community. Since bats were a major source of protein among local residents, they were widely hunted by villagers before the epidemic, which brought them into contact with the virus (Leroy et al. 2009).

To some extent, the first case of Ebola implicitly tied to human migration in West Africa was observed during a minor outbreak in Ivory Coast in 1994. A Swiss scientist conducting research among dead chimpanzees in Taï National Park was infected by the virus and subsequently evacuated to Switzerland, where she received treatment and later recovered from the disease (Georges et al. 1999). Another implicit case was that associated with a localized Ebola outbreak in Liberia in 1996. In this case, there was a confirmed case of Ebola in the village of Gozon in Ivory Coast, located fifteen miles from the border with Liberia, involving a refugee fleeing the war in Liberia who was admitted to the village's health facility (United Nations [UN] 1995). As in the 2013 epidemic in West Africa, the 2001–2003 Ebola epidemic in Gabon and the DRC was also traced to a border region straddling both countries. Possibly as a result of localized population movements, the ensuing epidemic resulted in the death of at least sixty-two people across both countries (Rouquet et al. 2005).

One of the most definitive cases of human-to-human transmission of Ebola tied to international migration was that associated with the first case of Ebola observed in South Africa. In 1996, a South African nurse became ill and was suspected of having encephalitis, although subsequent tests showed that she had, in fact, contracted Ebola. Her infection was traced to an interaction with a sick doctor, who had earlier arrived in South Africa from Libreville in Gabon. Tests conducted after he was discharged showed that he had recently developed the antibody for the Ebola virus (WHO 1996).

None of these prior Ebola outbreaks generated the same degree of global anxiety as that tied to the recent West African epidemic. These more recent concerns were the product of at least two factors. The first was the influence of the global media in communicating information on the deadly nature of the virus and its ease of transmission between persons. In the process, global audiences became aware that, because of Ebola's high viral load, it was easy for contact with the disease to result in an infection within a very short period (Brantly, Brantly, and Thomas 2015). Based on this knowledge, it became easy to consider the possibility that Ebola-infected travelers could be silent agents of transmission of the virus. The second explanation was that the structural influences shaping the risks of the international transmission of the disease were better developed compared to those associated with prior epidemics. In other words, this was the first time that an Ebola outbreak had occurred in densely populated settlements with advanced transportation links that could connect them to cities in other regions.

Immigrant Communities and Disease Epidemics

After the death of Thomas Duncan in Dallas, the backlash against African immigrants was based on the assumption that they were infected with a disease that could be easily transmitted to others. However, this assumption understates what we know from the evidence on immigrant health. Compared to native-born populations, immigrants, including those from Africa, are usually in much better health (Cunningham et al. 2008; Reed et al. 2012; Singh and Miller 2004; Vang and Elo 2013). Yet, their exposure to diverse disease environments implies that their epidemiological profiles can reflect their complex history of exposure to various disease pathogens. Apart from these pathogens, the residential circumstances of immigrants also have implications for their disease etiology and the ways in which host communities respond to them during health crises. This is particularly the case for immigrants who live in disadvantaged socioeconomic contexts, because these contexts can increase their susceptibility to adverse health conditions and their vulnerability to stigma.

Such adverse conditions have played a critical role in shaping the experiences of immigrants during epidemics in the United States. During the 1892 typhus fever epidemic in New York, they were responsible for the outbreak of the disease among Russian Jewish immigrants who had recently arrived in the city (Markel 1999). Squalid conditions in the boardinghouses where they lived created an environment that accentuated their susceptibility to a disease incubated under the equally squalid conditions on the ship on which they had arrived. On their voyage on the MSS *Massilia*, they lived in unsanitary conditions, ate rotten food, and were severely malnourished. Conditions only worsened within the first few weeks of their arrival in New York due to a typhus fever outbreak, which was one of several that occurred in the city during the nineteenth century.

Public reactions to the epidemic were instructive of how host societies have since responded to immigrant communities during outbreaks of disease. First, there was backlash against Russian Jewish immigrants driven by the assumption that they were actively involved in transmitting the infection across the city (Markel 1999). Capitalizing on this backlash, some members of Congress even used the epidemic as a springboard for pushing new legislation to ban the immigration of Russian Jews. A second type of reaction was that observed by public health officials. They decided to intervene using policies that were ostensibly geared toward tamping down public fears and controlling the spread of the disease. Russian Jewish immigrant neighborhoods were thus quarantined; however, this only served to reinforce the public perception of their community as a significant threat to public health.

Anti-immigrant backlash and municipal health interventions are now among the most critical elements expected to be observed in immigrant communities during epidemics. The former is particularly consequential for the lived experiences of immigrants when their communities are perceived to be tied to the sources of epidemics abroad. One such link was observed during the 1892 cholera epidemic in New York. Toward the end of the typhus fever epidemic that same year, reports began to emerge that there was a massive cholera epidemic occurring in Russia (Markel 1999). These reports increased concerns that the disease would be transmitted to the United States by Russian Jewish immigrants, because they were still arriving in the country in large numbers. In late 1892, these fears were confirmed with the spread of the disease to the United States by Russian travelers arriving in New York. Fears about the possible spread of cholera preceded the outbreak of the disease in the city; as a result, the start of the outbreak was marked by a predictable rise in anti-immigrant sentiments (Merkel 1995, 1999). Less than a decade later, the link between epidemics and anti-immigrant backlash was reinforced after the start of the bubonic plague in Honolulu and San Francisco. Originating in the southwest region of China a few years earlier, the plague subsequently spread to Hong Kong and Canton before it reached the United States (Barde 2004). After the outbreak occurred in Honolulu and San Francisco, the backlash was immediate, and in some cases it involved the burning of houses of infected persons.

More than a century later, the construction of immigrants as threats to public health remained an integral part of the public response to epidemics in many Western societies. During the SARS outbreak in the United States and Canada, for example, the main targets of backlash were Chinese immigrant communities. Concerns about the virus negatively affected Chinese-owned businesses, as their clients took steps to avoid any contact with recent immigrants from Asia (Blendon et al. 2003). More importantly, the perceived threat of SARS was racialized in a way that extended the stigma of the disease to other emigrants from Asia. In New York's Chinatown, the perceived threat posed by the "Chinese" disease increased as rumors spread about the apparent death of a well-known Asian restaurant owner who actually turned out to be Vietnamese (Eichelberger 2007). These reactions were not just being observed in the United States. In Canada, patronage of restaurants in Toronto's Chinatown declined as the public became apprehensive of what they considered a new Chinese disease (Keil and Ari 2006). Similarly, many Asian-origin immigrants were harassed and ostracized, while some hotels refused to accommodate guests from China (Leung 2008).

Racialized public reactions toward immigrants during epidemics usually stand in stark contrast to the corresponding reactions to native-born groups that are similarly affected during these periods. Accordingly, while Chinese-owned businesses were being destroyed during the bubonic plague in San Francisco, White-owned businesses in Chinese communities were left undisturbed (Barde 2004). Analyses of public responses to epidemics in Canada across two periods have found similar differences. Jones (2005) suggests, for example, that compared to the anti-Chinese backlash observed during the SARS epidemic, the public response to native-born communities tied to the 1918–1919 influenza pandemic was more muted.*

What we know about the social response to immigrant communities during epidemics therefore suggests that these responses are characterized by at least three specific patterns. First, there is the stigmatization of groups that are perceived to have the most direct links with the foreign origins of the disease. This stigmatization is sometimes more intense when fears about the spread of disease from abroad precede the outbreak of the disease on US soil. Second, the backlash toward immigrants is subsequently racialized. In the absence of objective ways of identifying persons infected

---

* This, he suggests, stems from the fact that the 1918–1919 influenza pandemic in Winnipeg was directly tied to a group of twenty-three Canadian soldiers returning home from World War I while also being traced to relatively wealthy neighborhoods in the province.

with the disease, ethnicity, racial minority status, and national origins be-come the major bases used to identify the possible targets of stigma.* Fi-nally, the immigrant groups that often receive the brunt of the backlash tend to live in contexts of socioeconomic disadvantage. This was as true of the Russian Jews in New York in 1892 as it was of the poor community in Dallas where Thomas Duncan lived before he died of Ebola in 2014.

Stigma, Race, and Infectious Disease

It took about two weeks from the start of the West African Ebola epi-demic for the effects of stigma to become apparent. The first evidence of this came in the experiences of Emile Ouamouno's father, Etienne, who was one of the few people fortunate enough to have survived the initial outbreak of the virus. Life became more difficult for him not so much because of the loss of his son but because of how locals reacted after the virus was traced to his family. Approximately one-third of Meliandou's residents left for other communities because they believed the Ouamouno family had brought a curse to their village (Faul 2014). To be sure, how-ever, the early signs of the stigmatization of the Ouamouno family emerged very shortly after the start of the outbreak. Mourners who attended Ebola-related funerals in the village refused to follow the local custom of eating food provided for them by the bereaved families.

Shortly thereafter, Meliandou itself became a source of stigma. Resi-dents in nearby communities blamed the village for being the source of the lethal epidemic, and the consequences of this stigma negatively affected Meliandou's economy. Although farmers from the village typically sold their crops at the large markets in nearby Guéckédo, there was a signifi-cant drop in demand for these crops after the start of the outbreak (Beukes 2014). Yet, these were not isolated incidents. The stigmatization of Ebola survivors has also been observed in other African communities where prior Ebola epidemics have occurred. After the 2001 Ebola outbreak in Gulu, Uganda, for example, survivors were ostracized by members of their community during visits to local markets and boreholes, as well as during

---

* This was also observed in the early 1800s, when Irish immigrants were blamed for spreading cholera and, toward the end of the century, when tuberculosis was considered a Jewish disease (Kraut 2010).

walks in their neighborhoods (Hewlett and Amola 2003). Similarly, survivors of the 1995 Ebola epidemic in Kikwit in the DRC developed a distinct fear of being abandoned by their families as a result of the stigma of the virus (De Roo et al 1998). These reactions are not surprising, because stigmas targeting people associated with disease are as old as the history of disease itself. They have defined public reactions to people with epilepsy for more than four thousand years (Keusch et al. 2006). This fear-based response to disease is driven by the belief that individuals affected by an ailment possess specific characteristics that are harmful to society.

The experiences of Ebola survivors in Meliandou further highlight the strong connection among stigma, prejudice, and discrimination. Stigma and prejudice in particular are associated with processes that trigger negative reactions and stereotypes that facilitate the process of social rejection (Phelan et al. 2008). Significantly, however, there is a defined social order in which these reactions are observed. More powerful and socially connected groups are more likely to be shielded from these consequences, while socially vulnerable and powerless groups are more likely to be exposed to them. For these reasons, the targets of stigma during epidemics are most often members of minority groups already subjected to systematic patterns of prejudice and discrimination, even before the outbreak of disease.

Historical accounts are replete with evidence underscoring the relationship between minority status and disease-related stigma in US society. However, no group exemplifies the strength of this relationship as much as US-born Blacks, whose experiences with stigma extend back to the time of slavery. Back then, public perceptions of the health of Black slaves were characterized by a belief in their reliance on quackery and their use of strange elements such as snakes and chicken heads as a basis for promoting good health (Postell 1951). In the decades following the end of slavery, this stigmatization of Black health continued. White Americans with the smallest trace of Negro ancestry were assumed to be stricken by hideous diseases or to have the potential to contract dangerous infections that would afflict them with ailments later in life (Myrdal et al. 1964). This continued stigmatization of Black health had several consequences. One was the preference for White blood over Black blood during blood transfusions; another was the perception that persons affected by the sickle cell gene, which mostly affects Blacks, needed to be tattooed on their foreheads (Wailoo 2006). African descent in early American society was thus associated with a double burden of stigma. It was stigmatized based on the presumption of Black racial inferiority and on the basis of its association with the use of exotic practices.

While the end of slavery ended the large-scale arrival of Black Africans to the United States, the 1965 immigration reforms paved the way for a new wave of voluntary immigration from Africa. Yet, this shift occurred in a context where the stigmatization of people of African descent continued to persist. By the 1980s, for example, the start of the human immunodeficiency virus (HIV) / acquired immune deficiency syndrome (AIDS) epidemic ushered in a new era in which US-born Blacks and Haitians of African descent were the principal groups stigmatized as carriers of the infectious disease (Deacon et al. 2005). This stigmatization of Black bodies was institutionalized when the Centers for Disease Control and Prevention (CDC) adopted a new strategy for differentiating between high- and low-risk groups (Devine et al. 1999). After thirty-four Haitian immigrants were diagnosed with Kaposi's sarcoma, a cancer often found among individuals infected with HIV, the CDC officially classified Haitian immigrants as a high-risk group; that is, they were among the most likely to be infected with the disease (CDC 1982; Curran and Jaffe 2011; Marc et al. 2010).

African immigrants arriving in the United States in the late 1980s were similarly stigmatized. Responding to the growing HIV/AIDS epidemic in sub-Saharan Africa, the Food and Drug Administration (FDA) instituted a ban that made it impossible for Africans to donate blood (Fairchild and Tynan 1994). However, this ban was issued despite the fact that there were available tests to determine whether prospective donors were infected with the virus. The decision was rationalized using arguments that invoked long-held stereotypes about the health of Africans, seeing them as immigrants who had large numbers of sexual partners and were widely involved in prostitution (Lambert 1990). In subsequent decades, the social context in which such stereotypes prevail has largely remained unchanged. Evidence suggests that perceptions of African immigrant health are still influenced by stereotypes that consider their origin societies as primitive, distant, and ravaged by disease (Iheduru 2013).

Recent epidemics linked to African immigrant communities provide us with new opportunities for observing how immigrant status and racial stereotypes are used in the construction of threats to public health. As the historical evidence demonstrates, the intersection of these factors has had a consistent influence on public reactions toward immigrant communities during health crises. A central characteristic of these periods is the racialization of disease using stereotypes and stigmas to create a dichotomy between us and them (Devine et al. 1999). During the SARS epidemic, for example, the construction of Chinese immigrants as outsiders was reinforced using popular stereotypes that considered their communities as places where people feasted on wild animals such as civet cats (Keil and Ali 2006).

After the start of the Ebola crisis in Dallas, stereotypes were similarly incorporated into the process of racializing the disease and identifying appropriate targets of stigma. The index case, Thomas Duncan, was from an exotic region where people consumed strange animals, such as bats and various types of bush meat. After his death, the parallels between the emerging patterns of stigmatization and those used to stigmatize the health of Black slaves became more striking. Accordingly, the presumed threat posed by African immigrants was racialized by some commentators, who used the prevalence of non-Western burial practices in Africa to argue that these immigrants bring their otherness with them when they arrive in American communities (Grey and Devlin 2015). The root of these fears was the connection between the transmission of the Ebola virus and African cultural practices such as the washing of corpses. Rather than situating these practices in the context of the lack of modern mortuaries in rural Africa, however, they were frequently deployed in the construction of stigma during the Ebola crisis in Dallas.

Before the Dallas crisis, similar African stereotypes were deployed in the public reaction to the first Ebola-related event observed among immigrants in North America. As was true of Thomas Duncan's experience in Texas, a young lady traveling from Africa arrived in Hamilton, Ontario, Canada, and was subsequently admitted to a hospital after showing symptoms of illness. As far as the public was concerned, her case was suspicious because she was from the DRC, where the Ebola virus was first identified. Also concerning was the fact that her symptoms were quite similar to those of Ebola. To make things worse, reports emerged that she was "bleeding from several sites on her body" (Adeyanju and Oriola 2010, 34), although this misrepresented the fact that the sick patient was menstruating at the time that she was admitted to the hospital. Reacting to these events, many members of the media concluded that she was an Ebola patient while emphasizing her status as an outsider from a continent marked by the disease (Murdocca 2003). Widespread fears about the African who supposedly brought Ebola to Canada ensued, which some scholars maintained were driven by stereotypes of Africans as primitive savages (Adeyanju and Neverson 2007). After the presumed Ebola case proved to be unfounded, perceptions of the threat posed by African immigrants continued to prevail. However, they were reframed in the process of emphasizing the potential threat of a true Ebola epidemic in Canada as globalization increased (Adeyanju and Neverson 2007).

Notwithstanding the significance of previous studies, most accounts of the deployment of stigma in immigrant communities during epidemics ignore the ways in which stigma can influence social interactions among immigrants themselves. This one-dimensional treatment of stigma understates the variation in immigrants' cultural practices, beliefs about illness, and strategies used to mitigate exposure to disease. As Etienne Ouamouno's experience in Meliandou suggests, fear-based reactions are incorporated into the ways in which people respond to disease, even in African immigrant origin societies.

Beliefs about disease developed before migration are, therefore, critical in determining how immigrants respond to illness and disease in their own communities. Studies have thus found that even immigrant groups that have historically been stigmatized by the public during epidemics continue to maintain stigmas of their own. Chinese immigrants have stigmas associated with dementia, HIV, and hepatitis (Cotler et al. 2012; Kang et al. 2005; Liu et al. 2008); Russian Jewish immigrants have mental health stigmas (Brodsky 1988); and African immigrants tend to have stigmas about diseases such as HIV/AIDS, hypertension, and depression (Venters and Gany 2011).

Epidemics and the Incorporation of Immigrants into Society

A major reason we should care about immigrants' experiences during epidemics is that they reflect the influence of larger social forces that shape their incorporation into society. To begin with, the presence of perceived boundaries between immigrants and native-born populations during epidemics is a clear reflection that immigrants' incorporation into society is incomplete. At the same time, immigrants' ability to respond effectively to epidemics is largely affected by the degree to which they are incorporated into their communities. Sociologists are at the forefront of identifying the factors that determine the success of immigrant incorporation processes. These factors include institutions, social stratification systems, and generational status, and they have been used in the development of several perspectives predicting the likely pathways along which incorporation processes are likely to unfold.

Drawing from the experiences of European immigrants arriving in the early 1900s, the earliest perspectives underscored the disadvantages of first-generation immigrants that limit their degree of integration into society (Alba and Nee 1997; Gordon 1961, 1964). For the most part, these disadvantages stem from limited access to opportunities and culturally distinctive factors such as the use of mother tongues that help to reinforce their status as outsiders. Like many African immigrants in Dallas or Russian Jews during the 1892 cholera epidemic, first-generation immigrants are incorporated in a process defined by their limited familiarity with US social systems, inadequate access to social networks, and residence in poor communities. Some of these characteristics also increase their vulnerability to the negative consequences of stigma during epidemics. From this conventional assimilation perspective, however, the disadvantages experienced by immigrants often decline as generational status increases (Alba and Nee 1997; Greenman and Xie 2008). In other words, the descendants of first-generation immigrants are likely to experience greater levels of social integration and therefore are more likely to be able to better navigate the influence of negative social forces.

The increasing diversity of immigrants that followed the 1965 immigration reforms revealed many of the limitations of the conventional assimilation perspective. Compared to their White European counterparts, most descendants of non-European immigrants failed to experience the improved social outcomes predicted by the conventional assimilation perspective. To address these new realities, the segmented assimilation perspective was developed to highlight the influence of structural factors such

as contexts of reception, community resources, and systems of racial stratification on the social incorporation of immigrants (Portes and Zhou 1993;
Zhou 1997). In terms of contexts of reception, it maintained that refugee
groups generally have more favorable outcomes because they arrive in
more receptive contexts than other immigrants. Accordingly, their vulnerabilities are mitigated by their access to various types of social services
and assistance provided by the government. Community resources are expected to promote positive immigrant incorporation experiences largely
because co-ethnic communities tend to have strong institutions that provide them with resources and the social capital needed for advancement.
Another set of influences emphasized by the segmented assimilation perspective is that associated with systems of racial stratification. Immigrants
from racial groups that have historically faced high levels of discrimination are often the most likely to experience negative incorporation outcomes (Portes and Zhou 1993). In part, this is because they tend to face
limited prospects of social acceptance and have frequent encounters with
racial prejudice and discrimination.

Scholarly analysis of the Ebola crisis in Dallas is important because it
allows us to observe how the interplay of contexts of reception, community resources, and racial minority status affected the lives of immigrants
during a major public health event. African immigration to the city, and
much of the United States, has partly been driven by a surge in the immigration of refugees (Kent 2007). These include refugees from countries
such as Somalia and Ethiopia, as well as their counterparts from Liberia
and Sierra Leone, two of the three countries that were at the epicenter of
the West African Ebola epidemic. As a central area for refugee settlement,
Dallas also hosts several institutions that provide various types of specialized resources to refugees. In addition, the growth in African settlement
in the city has been accompanied by major increases in the availability
of ethnic community resources. These include a rich collection of ethnic
churches, businesses, and niche organizations that serve the professional,
social, and economic needs of an African immigrant clientele.

Nevertheless, accumulating evidence indicates that race is a significant
barrier to the social incorporation of African immigrants. Like US-born
Blacks, they have frequent encounters with racial profiling and job discrimination, and are often the targets of racial slurs (Guenther et al. 2011).

In fact, African immigrant experiences with the disadvantage of racial minority status are so compelling that they appear to outweigh the benefits
of a favorable mode of incorporation typically observed among refugees
(Ali 2011).

The Ebola crisis in Dallas allows us to answer new questions about
whether the social forces that influence African immigrant incorporation
also shaped their experiences with the backlash received from the public
during the health crisis. Moreover, the crisis provides an opportunity for
investigating how factors that contributed to negative immigrant experiences differed from those that generated positive responses. At the same
time, it allows us to observe the extent to which ethnic institutions were
able to buffer the effects of stigma directed at Africans. Accounts from
previous epidemics suggest, for example, that positive contexts of reception and strong immigrant institutions are not always able to mitigate the
effects of anti-immigrant backlash. Refugees are thus stigmatized during
disease outbreaks despite the fact that they go through systematic health
screenings before arriving in the United States (Dellplain 2012). Furthermore, we have learned from the SARS epidemic that ethnic institutions
that are among the major providers of community resources can themselves be the targets of stigma. They represented the very symbols of the
racialized threat constructed by the public and were largely undermined
by the backlash against the Chinese.

Immigrant destinations such as Dallas further provide us with opportunities for exploring the implications of racial and ethnic minority status
for immigrant experiences during epidemics. Much of the evidence from
prior epidemics underscores the significance of race and ethnicity for the
construction of stigma. However, this perspective can be limiting, because
it fails to consider how immigrants themselves view the role of race in determining their experiences during epidemics. In addition, it ignores their
agency in countering the narrative of victimhood that frequently charac-
terizes the analysis of epidemics.

The Ebola Crisis in Dallas and New Perspectives on the Experiences of Immigrants

Drawing from the experiences of African immigrants in Dallas, therefore, this book provides new insights into the social implications of global

epidemics for immigrant communities abroad. A central part of this process is the development of a complex narrative that demonstrates how fear, racialized stigma, and agency are fundamental to understanding the diverse types of community responses that were observed after the death of Thomas Duncan. Exploiting the fact that the Dallas crisis occurred at a time of unprecedented globalization, this book also examines how the global dissemination of news about the epidemic fueled fears about the consequences of contact with infected persons. Apart from examining the dynamics of these fears, it underscores the agency that African immigrants demonstrated in their navigation of the consequences of stigma as well as their attempts to mitigate the consequences of the epidemic at its source in West Africa.

Two specific arguments are made to advance what we know about the social implications of epidemics. First, while recognizing the significance of minority status for construction of stigma during epidemics, I argue that the development and deployment of stigma in Dallas were more nuanced than what has typically been observed in previous studies. This argument does not ignore the historical role of anti-Black prejudice and African stereotypes in the construction of stigma. In fact, this role is underscored by situating the anti-African backlash within our understanding of the role of racial stratification in creating barriers to the incorporation experiences of African immigrants. While this way of understanding the development of stigma is important, it is nevertheless limiting. It minimizes the ways in which fears about the Ebola virus shaped the construction of stigma within the African immigrant community. Furthermore, it ignores the ways in which immigrants employ differences in national origins, ethnicity, and socioeconomic status in the deployment of these stigmas.

Moving beyond the narrative of victimhood used in the analysis of epidemics, the second argument is that immigrants are active participants in shaping the response to disease outbreaks tied to their communities. This argument highlights immigrants' agency in dealing with the negative consequences of epidemics while shifting attention away from the restricted focus on their experiences as victims. In the process, the larger responses of African immigrants during the crisis are analyzed from two complementary perspectives. The first is their response to the public backlash to

the crisis in Dallas, while the second is their response to the global consequences of the outbreak. As the analysis suggests, these global responses
were in many ways facilitated by their prior involvement in transnational
circuits of migration.

Much of the information used to make these arguments is taken from
qualitative data sources. The primary data source is a survey conducted
among key informants who lived or worked among African immigrants in
the Dallas area during the Ebola crisis.* These data came from two groups
of informants: leaders and representatives of African immigrant institutions, many of whom were directly involved in the response to the crisis
(86 percent),† and officials of humanitarian aid organizations and institutions that provided diverse services to African immigrants (e.g., refugees)
in Dallas (14 percent).‡ When they are discussed in the book, all key informants are given pseudonyms in order to preserve their anonymity.§
Similarly, pseudonyms are also used for the immigrant organizations mentioned in the book to further help to anonymize the key informants linked
with these organizations. Apart from information from key informants,
information was collected from participant observations conducted at
African immigrant community events (e.g., parties, church services, and
meetings) and in African-owned institutions such as restaurants and hair-
braiding salons. This strategy was used to develop insights on the dynamics of social interaction among African immigrants and to observe the
cultivation and deployment of various sources of social capital within the
community. In addition to these sources, supplementary information was
collected from government documents, public archives, and other public

* This survey was conducted between May and August 2016, almost two years after the
Ebola crisis in Dallas, and it targeted fifty key informants in the area.

† In a few cases, this group also included patrons of immigrant establishments and other
key informants recommended by African immigrant leaders. This subgroup of key informants accounted for less than 10 percent of the final sample.

‡ Leaders of organizations such as the International Rescue Committee, which provided
services to African refugees, were the only non-Africans interviewed in the survey. Many
African refugees could not be interviewed because they were not proficient in English.
These leaders were also involved in the response to the crisis.

§ The names of other major subjects in the book, including Thomas Duncan and Reverend Jesse Jackson, are not anonymized. Not only is their participation in the events associated with the crisis in Dallas found in public records, but they were also not interviewed
in the survey used in this book.

sources. The major sources of supplementary information include the Dallas Public Library, the Dallas Department of Public Health, and the archives of the *Dallas Morning News.*

Chapter 2 discusses the implications of globalization for how societies respond to epidemics. I argue that these implications are becoming more significant in the contemporary world, and that they provide a basis for understanding two sets of responses. The first set is represented by the negative responses of fear and blaming. As theories examining the relationship between epidemics and fear suggest, these responses are particularly salient in contexts of widespread ignorance and misinformation. While these responses are extensively discussed in previous studies, I contend that it is important to integrate a second set of responses—prosocial responses— into our understanding of community responses to epidemics. The most important of these prosocial responses are demonstrations of agency and displays of resilience. These prosocial responses, I reason, are important for understanding how communities develop counteractions to mitigate the negative consequences of epidemics.

Chapter 3 frames the contextual foundation upon which the book's core arguments are developed by describing the social organization of life in African immigrant communities in the Dallas area. This foundation is used as a basis for understanding the strengths and vulnerabilities of the social context in which African immigrants' experiences occur. In this chapter, I highlight African immigrants' specific pathways of immigration and settlement as well as the diverse ways in which they are incorporated into society. Some of the challenges they encounter during this process include racial discrimination, negative African stereotypes, and limited socioeconomic mobility among disadvantaged groups, such as refugees. Despite these challenges, I argue that life in the African immigrant community traditionally revolves around the provision of mutual support, bounded solidarity, and activities designed to help those in need. Most African immigrants, for example, have access to co-ethnic institutions that support the economic integration of families and the educational success of their children. These institutions further help families respond to emergencies and connect them to a wider network of resources in the Dallas metropolitan area. Significantly, these institutions also provide a major mechanism for transferring resources from Africans in Dallas to poor communities in their origin countries. I thus show in this chapter that co-ethnic institutions in the African community in Dallas amassed considerable experience in helping their members cope with crises, even before the start of the Ebola outbreak.

Chapter 4 focuses on immigrants from the three West African countries that were most affected by the epidemic to examine how they experienced the early consequences of the epidemic. Drawing from accounts of those who visited these countries during the outbreak, I argue that immigrants involved in transnational migration between Dallas and West Africa were the first residents of the city to be exposed to risks of contracting Ebola. To begin this argument, I describe why these immigrants chose to travel to these countries, after which I examine the innovative strategies they used to avoid being infected by the virus. I also give attention to responses of fear that began to emerge among those who remained in Dallas as they learned more about the virus. This knowledge had significant consequences, one of which was the stigmatization of Africans returning to the city from affected countries in Africa. I further claim that many Africans in Dallas experienced a double burden of the epidemic. The first was associated with the traumatic experiences of those who lost relatives to Ebola at home. These experiences were compounded by their inability to go back to Africa to participate in cultural processes of mourning. The second was their subsequent experiences in Dallas, especially those associated with the public backlash against Africans after the death of Thomas Duncan.

Chapter 5 uses the specific events surrounding the Ebola crisis in Dallas to illustrate how the death of Thomas Duncan provided a new basis for constructing Africans as threats to public health. It documents the diverse responses to his death in the city, which include responses of fear, blame, and anger. In the process, it contrasts the narratives of blame that had been developed by the public and the corresponding narratives used by African immigrants to understand the crisis. Particular attention is given to the debate concerning whether the perceived threat of Ebola-infected persons was racialized by comparing the backlash against Thomas Duncan and his family to the public response toward the two nurses infected by the virus while caring for Duncan in Dallas. Although many people suggest that negative public reaction to the death of Duncan was driven by racism, I contend that among African immigrants, the use of racial frameworks to understand his experiences was more complex.

Chapter 6 focuses on the public backlash against African immigrants in Dallas while demonstrating how the deployment of stigma differed from that found in the standard narratives on blame and stigma in previous studies. It underscores how racial stereotypes and African cultural symbols were incorporated into the construction of stigma and the various contexts in which these stigmas were deployed. Given the centrality of perceived Africanness in the development of these stigmas, I illustrate how the ensuing backlash was extended to immigrants from African countries who were removed from the source of the epidemic itself. Social interactions within the African community during the crisis also provide a basis for understanding the complexities of stigmatization processes. Accordingly, the chapter highlights how national origins and ethnic differences were deployed among Africans to stigmatize immigrants from countries affected by the epidemic. At the same time, I argue that the fear of Ebola was so prevalent in some sections of the African community that stigma was deployed as a way of mitigating the Ebola threat, even among immigrants with similar national origins.

Much of chapter 7 is used to examine the demonstrations of agency and displays of resilience among African immigrants in responding to the crisis. I demonstrate in this chapter how co-ethnic institutions and community resources that traditionally supported the incorporation of African immigrants were used to organize two types of deliberative responses. The first was the response to the crisis in Dallas. I maintain that these responses were observed at the personal as well as at the institutional level. The individual responses were reflected in the wide range of strategies employed by Africans to control the spread of the disease. They also included measures to cope with stigma, including identifying themselves using different nationalities, as they navigated interactions with the larger community of Dallas. Institutional responses involved the structured attempts made by African immigrant institutions to counter the public backlash. Second, and more importantly, the I examine immigrants' responses to the crisis in the African countries that were at the center of the epidemic. I demonstrate how African immigrants mobilized immigrant resources and activated their wider networks in Dallas to help provide relief and humanitarian assistance to the most affected countries.

Chapter 8 draws parallels between the typical experiences of immigrant communities in prior epidemics and those of African immigrants during the Ebola crisis in Dallas. Beyond these parallels, I systematically highlight the unique lessons that we can learn from African immigrant experiences. One of these is the dual significance of globalization for immigrants during epidemics. As their experiences demonstrate, transnational processes expose immigrants to the negative consequences of epidemics abroad while at the same time providing the global connections needed to conduct an international response to epidemics. Drawing from the responses of African immigrants to the crisis in Dallas, I also call for the expansion of studies on immigrant community resources that specifically address the diverse ways in which they act to buffer immigrants during periods of crisis. This will require a greater appreciation of the role of immigrant agency in responding to these events. The chapter concludes by reinforcing the argument that immigrants are not passive observers indifferent to the negative consequences of stigma during epidemics but are active participants who can shape the narrative of their experiences and alleviate the lives of those who experience the adverse consequences of epidemics in other parts of the world.

2 Fear, Blame, and the Social Response to Epidemics

Epidemics are watershed moments that attract a collective response from society. When they create an international emergency, the scale of this response is extensive and affected by factors such as the perceived threat of disease, the actions of health institutions, and the strategies used for containment (Lau et al. 2003; Van Damme and Van Lerberghe 2004). Responses developed to address the consequences of these emergencies are fundamental to understanding the relationship between globalization and disease. On the one hand, the relationship between the two is affected by mechanisms such as the mobility of people and services, which can affect the capacity of societies to respond to epidemics (Fidler 2001; Zimmet 2000). On the other hand, these same mechanisms can accelerate the transmission of information that promotes the spread of fear and the development of stigmas across international borders (Rübsamen et al. 2015; Ungar 1998).

Within countries, local communities are the most immediate contexts in which such responses are developed. Consequently, they are frequently used to situate studies on responses to epidemics that focus on diseases originating within their borders or in other parts of the world. Each of these origins represents a context that can create an international epidemic on its own. However, the origins of the Ebola crisis in Dallas were different. Indeed, the crisis was created by disease outbreaks that originated both within the city's boundaries and in other countries.

Before examining the specific responses observed in Dallas, it is important to understand the broader context in which such responses are typically developed. For example, how do communities usually respond to the threat of epidemics? What factors affect how these responses are initiated?

In what ways can the social response to epidemics undermine or enhance the welfare of groups others blame for the spread of disease?

Critical to the process of answering these questions is the need to recognize the role of globalization in transforming the social structure of the very communities in which these responses occur. Like Dallas, many American cities have experienced these transformations as they have adjusted to the settlement of immigrants from an increasing number of countries. As these immigrant settlements are established, so too are social and economic inequalities accentuated, while new traditions are incorporated into the cultural fabric of their communities. The establishment of these new immigrant groups creates new challenges for local authorities. For example, it forces them to develop ways of thinking about how to improve public health. Moreover, it requires that they carefully manage differences in the cultural and social experiences of immigrants and natives. Perceptions of these differences can vary in these new destinations. As a result, these differences can represent fault lines that can negatively affect social cohesion or can provide opportunities for building coalitions for community development.

Responses developed to address the health challenges of immigrants do not always bridge these differences successfully. Instead, they fall along a wide spectrum. At one end is the development of culturally responsive strategies that address the health needs of immigrants. These include modifications to the operations of healthcare providers and the provision of cultural sensitivity training to medical staff (Dysart-Gale 2007; Williamson and Harrison 2010). At the other end are responses that exploit the cultural attributes of immigrants to develop health stereotypes and that create structural barriers that limit their access to essential services (Reitmanova and Gustafson 2008).

When epidemics are linked to immigrant communities, the stakes for local residents are significant. To make things worse, if the epidemic is linked with a deadly disease, local residents frequently develop an urge to respond by using strategies that negatively affect the welfare of immigrants. Most previous studies of such epidemics, therefore, focus on negative social responses that affect the lives of immigrants. However, these accounts are inadequate, and they are inconsistent with what we know about the wide range of responses observed during periods of crisis and other types of emergencies.

One way to move beyond this limited approach is to provide a balanced account of social responses to epidemics that capture two sets of responses. The first includes responses that negatively target communities affected by these events, and the most common of these are expressions of fear and the tendency to blame. Both responses are associated with mass reactions of panic and are driven by a desire to avoid the fatal consequences of infection (Alcabes 2009; Covey 2001). The second set includes responses that are prosocial, chief of which are demonstrations of agency and displays of resilience (DeWitte et al. 2016; Ruger 2007). Rather than capitulating to the urge to react negatively, these responses help to counter the adverse consequences of epidemics.

This two-pronged approach is important, and it provides a basis for developing a more objective perspective on the social implications of epidemics. It also broadens the analysis beyond a focus on groups who face negative reactions and the backlash against their communities. When these accounts are balanced by the examination of prosocial responses, it becomes possible to extend the analysis to focus on other actors, including local residents who work to help communities recover from the social disorder created by epidemics.

Fear as a Response to Disease

Fear is an emotional response to the threat of harm rooted in the desire for self-preservation and is extensively studied in the health and social sciences (Tudor 2003; Witte and Allen 2000). In recent years, however, increased attention has been given to the importance of fear as a social response to globalization (Body-Gendrot 2012; Keohane 2002; Pain 2009). From this perspective, fear is understood as a response to global events such as acts of terrorism, international financial crises, and environmental disasters (Pain 2009). These events are associated with reactions of panic in one part of the world that are easily transmitted to another. Moreover, the increased attention given to the threat they pose to society has resulted in the development of a metanarrative of fear that is defined by its focus on concerns about global security (Pain 2009).

Studies on the fear of disease have a longer history than this recent focus on security, and they provide extensive documentation of how societies have responded to the threat of disease extending as far back as the medieval period (Alcabes 2009; Van Damme and Van Lerberghe 2000). Between the thirteenth and eighteenth centuries, for example, there were several notable cases of fear-related responses to the spread of disease in Europe. These fears resulted from the belief that epidemics were consequences of sin and the actions of vengeful deities, and were accompanied by the adoption of various strategies of appeasement (Delumeau 1990). Accordingly, the spread of the Black Death and the subsequent deaths of millions were accompanied by the mass confession of sins and a public search for forgiveness (Alcabes 2009). Expressions of fear were also among the most common responses to the smallpox epidemic in England in the 1800s. In the ensuing crisis, for example, churchyards were filled with corpses, while the spread of the virus tormented those alive with fears that caused them to shudder (Barquet and Domingo 1997). Such fears of disease are not restricted to cases where death is an immediate consequence of infection. These fears have been found to be pervasive when the prospects of death are less daunting, if the morbidity consequences of infection are generally believed to be irreversible (Brandt 1988; Covey 2001; Gussow and Tracy 1970).

In more recent decades, diseases at the center of global epidemics have generated fears that are transmitted along patterns dictated by progress toward completion of the epidemiological transition. As previous research indicates, epidemiological transitions describe changes in cause of death profiles over time that usually involve a shift from infectious to chronic diseases as the dominant causes of death (Omran 2005). While most Western countries have completed these transitions, poor, developing countries are still in the earlier stages of transition and consequently account for disproportionately large numbers of deaths from infectious diseases (Lozano et al. 2012). As a result of these differences, Western fears about the global threat of epidemics are informed by the expectation that diseases transmitted during these events are most likely to originate in poor, developing countries (Jones et al. 2008; Morens and Fauci 2013). In other words, developing countries are seen as breeding grounds for emerging infectious diseases such as Ebola as well as reemerging infectious diseases that are becoming more resistant to antibiotics (Morens and Fauci 2013; Morens et al. 2004).

As it turns out, global epidemics originating in developing countries do not occur as frequently as is commonly perceived. But, this has not curtailed the use of these contexts to advance a narrative of fear in the West. It is embedded in discourses that highlight the threat of biological agents that could be weaponized for mass destruction, such anthrax and smallpox (Morens et al. 2004). Not surprisingly, the Ebola virus prominently features in these discourses because of its presumed potential for exploitation by terrorists (Cunha 2002; Polesky and Bhatia 2003). Scientists dispute such claims by arguing that the virus is too contagious for terrorists to weaponize it (Cunha 2002). Yet, the fear of Ebola remains a central tool used in the construction of the threat of terrorism, as demonstrated in fear-based claims that maintain that terrorists could disperse samples of Ebola-infected fluids in US public places (Thiessen 2014). The social production of the fear of viruses is important; it suggests that there is a critical mass of people in the West who anticipate future epidemics in their local communities caused by viruses from developing countries.

A nuanced extension to this perspective is provided by Ungar (1998) in his work on hot crises in the United States. Based on his examination of the fears generated by the 1995 Ebola epidemic in Zaire, he argues that there is a fascination with deadly diseases in the United States that predisposes Americans to reactions of grassroots panic. Before the epidemic, for example, the fear of Ebola was popularized by the book *The Hot Zone* (Preston 1995), which describes the chaos caused by the virus in a military facility in Virginia. This fear of deadly viruses is not only promoted by literary accounts but also by cinematic representations of epidemics in movies and on TV shows. The result of this, according to Ungar, is that microbial contagion is now incorporated into how globalization is understood, with Ebola specifically seen "as an exotic jumper virus from an unknown host in the rainforest of Africa" (1998, 46). This fear of Ebola, and its association with a biological apocalypse originating in Africa, continued after the 1995 Ebola epidemic, and it was observed in the United States just before the start of the more recent crisis in Dallas (Belvedere 2014; Ungar 1998).

By themselves, epidemics in developing countries are unlikely to generate global expressions of fear. These responses draw on the latent fear of deadly viruses in other countries and are advanced by other important mechanisms. The most important of these is modern telecommunications technology. This technology makes it possible to transmit real-time information from the most remote locations in the world to a global audience. Today, the operations of global media organizations help to advance the fear of epidemics more than at any time in human history (Rübsamen et al. 2015; Ungar 1998). The information they provide is then used by pundits who describe to global audiences how these events should be interpreted.

This role of the media in framing threat perceptions is well documented in previous studies (Ridout et al. 2008; Scheufele 1999). These accounts indicate that media reports can leave very little room for ambiguity on how global threats should be interpreted. For example, reporters can structure coverage of the threat of global warming in a way that promotes the need for collective action (Olausson 2009). Furthermore, reports indicate that coverage on the nuclear threat from North Korea among news organizations can be framed to reflect the foreign policy objectives of the countries where they are located (Dai and Hyun 2010). Similar influences have been found in the reporting of global epidemics. For instance, during the SARS epidemic the disease was framed by media organizations in the United Kingdom in ways that emphasized its potential to become a deadly killer (Wallis and Nerlich 2005). Similarly, media coverage of the threat of the H5N1 virus (avian influenza) was framed to convey various messages ranging from those that were alarmist to those providing assurances of containment (Ungar 2008).

Ultimately, the media's promotion of fear during infectious disease epidemics leads to increased feelings of personal vulnerability. Exposure to TV news coverage during the avian flu epidemic was thus positively associated with individual concerns about the possibility of flu infection (Van den Bulck and Custers 2009). Media coverage of the West African Ebola epidemic in Germany similarly led to an increased fear of infection by the virus among Germans (Rübsamen et al. 2015). However, these fears were not just observed in Germany. They were also witnessed in other world regions, including Asia, South America, and North America, demonstrating the long reach of fear outside the boundaries of the origins of epidemics (Monson 2017; Sacramento and Machado 2015).

Blaming and Stigma

A second response to epidemics is the blaming of those suspected of transmitting the disease (Van Damme and Van Lerberghe 2000). Blaming leads to the development of stigmas, and both responses are related in the sense that the latter is usually a reaction to the former. Blaming arises from the need for attribution as well as a desire to identify the human causes of crises. In addition, it is driven by the desire to make sense of the negative consequences of presumably mysterious events, including epidemics (Nelkin and Gilman 1988). At the root of this quest for attribution is a desire to identify order in the midst of uncertainty. As such, the response of blaming people for the spread of disease is more prevalent in circumstances defined by the failure of medical science to provide a source of understanding and control (Nelkin and Gilman 1988).

A common practice used in the process of assigning blame during global epidemics is the identification of migrants as transmitters of disease. Such a practice can occur even when there are no explicit connections between migrants and the countries in which epidemics originate (Bigo 2002; Markel and Stern 2002). The evidence for such reactions is extensive. For example, in the sixteenth century immigrants were blamed for the spread of syphilis in Europe; however, the specific immigrant groups blamed for the disease varied across countries (Nelkin and Gilman 1988). Accordingly, French immigrants were blamed in Germany, Italians in France, and the Portuguese later in Japan (Nelkin and Gilman 1988). Several centuries later, in the 1890s, Jewish immigrants were blamed for the typhoid epidemic in New York, while in more recent years, immigrants have been blamed for the spread of tuberculosis in New Zealand and Africans for the spread of Ebola in the United States (Dionne and Seay 2015; Littleton et al. 2010).

Following the response of blaming is the development of stigmas, which were extensively discussed in the previous chapter. However, two remaining issues are worth noting. First, stigmas can emerge independently of the blaming process under conditions of extreme fear of disease. In recent years, for example, they have defined public reactions to diseases such as epilepsy, leprosy, and syphilis, in addition to conditions such as mental disorders (Brandt 1988; Gussow and Tracy 1970). In the process, stigmatized groups are seen from a reductionist perspective that generally links them with undesirable attributes considered harmful to society.

Second, how stigma is defined can affect the choice of groups used in the analysis of its implications. For instance, Goffman (1963) describes stigma as "an attribute that links a person to an undesirable stereotype, leading other people to reduce the bearer from a whole or usual person to a tainted, discounted one" (11). Similar definitions are found in other studies (Crocker et al. 1998; Stafford and Scott 1986) and, like that provided by Goffman, are developed to focus on the targets of stigma. This focus on the stigmatized group is, however, limited. As observed by Link and Phelan (2001), such conceptualizations emphasize the social response to *individuals* rather than the process by which *others* stigmatize individuals. The latter, they argued, is important for understanding the significance of discrimination and differentials in power in the production of stigmas, because it shifts attention from the targets of stigma to the producers of stigma. When this perspective is embraced, the analysis of stigma can be extended to a broader set of circumstances that include the co-occurrence of labeling, stereotyping, separating, status loss, and discrimination (Link and Phelan 2001).

This broader perspective is important for several reasons. It draws attention to the negative ways in which stigmas are experienced by individuals blamed for the spread of disease. It highlights the importance of the downstream consequences of blaming, which include a loss of status, and finally, it recognizes the importance of power differentials between groups that use blaming as a response to epidemics and groups blamed by their actions (Phelan, Link, and Dovidio 2008).

Agency, Health, and Epidemics

Demonstrations of agency during epidemics are quite distinct from negative social responses such as fear and blaming. Rather than focusing on reactions that accentuate the social disorder created by epidemics, they are concerned with the deliberate steps taken by individuals to address the consequences of these events. In short, agency recognizes that individuals have the ability to shape their responses based on their assessment of a possible set of actions. The concept has its origins in the Enlightenment period, during debates concerning the role of instrumental rationality or norm-based actions in the development of human freedoms (Emirbayer and Mische 1998). More recent conceptualizations of agency recognize the resourcefulness of people and their active involvement in the process of addressing the challenges they encounter (Elder 1994; Thompson 2001).

Agency is thus a major type of positive response observed during disasters, environmental shocks, and social crises (Adger et al. 2005; Brown and Westaway 2011). However, demonstrations of agency do not by themselves imply that the choice of action will be positive. Rather they allow for the possibility that the choices made by resourceful individuals during periods of crisis can have positive consequences. Many studies on human agency thus reflect this emphasis on choices that produce positive social change (Fukuda-Parr 2003; Ruger 2004). In so doing, they highlight the active involvement of people in shaping their destinies and refusing to be confined to the role of observers indifferent to the challenges they confront (Sen 1999). Studies that emphasize fear and blame as major social responses to epidemics ignore this human desire to make a difference. In part, this explains why few studies have attempted to articulate how stigmatized groups respond to the negative reactions that target them during epidemics to create positive change in the midst of tragedy.

This lack of research on these responses is surprising given the abundance of research on the relevance of agency for public health. Health scholars use the concept to describe the ability of individuals to pursue the goals they value and view it as a determinant of health functioning (Ruger 2007). In debates on the relative importance of personal responsibility and social responsibility for health outcomes, the importance of human agency is further used to underscore the relevance of the former compared to the latter (Minkler 1999). Communities can also demonstrate agency, and this involves taking deliberative actions to respond to health crises. Such actions, otherwise referred to as collective agency (Bandura 2004), reflect the ability of people to work together to accomplish change and to promote disease prevention.

Although systematic studies that examine the demonstration of agency as a response to epidemics are limited, historical studies provide scattered glimpses of the evolution of this response. These responses include community actions such as the performance of rituals and the offering of sacrifices, which are steps taken to ostensibly control the spread of disease

(Hays 2009). Recent studies in the medical sciences view the role of human agency in terms of either its significance for the inadvertent spread of disease or its absence in communities affected by epidemics (Arnold 1991; Phua and Lee 2005). This approach understates the importance of proactive actions to alter the course of epidemics and is considered by scholars to be a reflection of medical paternalism (Davis et al. 2011).

We know very little about how human agency is deployed by stigmatized communities, in part due to the assumption that their relative powerlessness undermines their ability to develop effective responses. Outside the health sciences, however, studies have shown that hierarchies of power are not necessarily constraints to the demonstration of agency. For instance, subaltern studies describe how low-status groups respond to crises related to colonialism by contesting experiences of stigma, power, domination, and subordination (Guha, Spivak, and Said 1988; Prakash 1994). Additionally, research on the work of trade unions and on minority groups during the civil rights era highlights the ability of the marginalized to resist hegemonic powers (Frost and Hoggett 2008; Gamson 1991). Rarely, however, are such perspectives employed in the examination of how low-status groups self-organize to contest the negative consequences of health crises (Frost and Hoggett 2008).

When epidemics have links to immigrant communities, this underlying assumption of indifference among the stigmatized can be problematic given what we know about the role of agency in the life of immigrants. Their ability to deploy agency across social contexts is extensively documented in studies showing that, rather than being isolated individuals who simply respond to social forces, immigrants actively seek to promote their well-being and that of their communities (Bakewell et al. 2012; Castles 2004; Gong et al. 2011). For example, at the individual level, immigrants demonstrate agency in the process of making the decision to migrate and navigating the social and legal challenges they encounter after arriving at their destinations (Gomberg-Muñoz 2010; Hoang 2011). At the same time, immigrants' use of community agency is seen in studies on their incorporation into new societies and their efforts to promote development in their countries of origin (Castles 2010). Therefore, regardless of whether immigrants are stigmatized, their use of agency is a central part of their repertoire for adapting to life in their host societies. As a result, they are unlikely to remain passive when faced by threats to public health that have negative implications for their welfare.

Resilience and Recovery

Agency is an important part of the larger range of prosocial responses to epidemics observed among individuals and communities. When correctly appropriated, it helps them rebound from crises, organize to prevent their reoccurrence, and emerge much stronger than they were before. This ability to overcome adversity is a product of resilience. Most public health studies highlight its importance as a positive determinant of health while linking it with characteristics such as optimism and perceived control, which facilitate recovery from life-threatening conditions (Chan et al. 2006; Plough et al. 2013).

Social disruptions created by epidemics provide a critical backdrop for understanding the significance of resilience. Following the massive loss of life during the Black Death in Europe, resilience was a determinant of how vulnerable groups recovered and was further instrumental in shaping the social transformations that later occurred across the continent (DeWitte et al. 2016). This protective and beneficial effect of resilience continues to be observed in more recent outbreaks of disease. For example, the influence of resilience was credited for the positive long-term health trajectory of persons infected with SARS during the 2003 outbreak in Hong Kong (Bonanno et al. 2008). After the start of the 2014 Ebola crisis in West Africa, resilience was also instrumental in helping Liberian communities develop innovative responses to the spread of the virus and successfully recover from the outbreak (Abramowitz et al. 2015).

Like agency, resilience can be observed at multiple levels of analysis. However, its influence is most frequently seen in the unfolding of individual responses to infection and disease (Hopwood and Treloar 2008). More importantly, resilient individuals stigmatized after contracting infectious diseases have been able to develop strategies to cope with rejection and to adjust to life within their communities. In other words, resilience can provide a crucial buffer that shields people from negative social responses that blame them for the spread of disease. Among groups, community resilience is another important response that can help in the recovery from crisis. This collective response is fostered by factors such as social connectedness, political leadership, and social solidarity (Nuwayhid et al. 2011; Plough et al. 2013). Both individual and community resilience can, however, act as part of a complex system that is useful for countering the negative social response to epidemics. For example, drawing from this perspective, DeWitte and colleagues (2016) illustrate the significance of this collective response in determining susceptibility to the bubonic plague in Europe and the reorganization of institutions during the process of recovery from the epidemic. This insight is important, and it can be employed in the study of the processes of recovery associated with contemporary public health emergencies.

Making Sense of the Response to Ebola in Dallas

Taken together, previous accounts of the social response to epidemics underscore the need to incorporate both antisocial and prosocial responses in analysis that aims to provide a comprehensive picture of the social implications of these events. Indeed, each specific type of response has additional implications for the examination of the response to Ebola in Dallas. Studies on expressions of fear, for example, suggest that there is a need to examine how the public narrative that was developed around the virus was influenced by concerns about threats to national security. However, they also suggest that the fear of Ebola may further be rooted in latent public perceptions of Africa as the origin of disease. It is important to investigate how these perceptions evolved during the crisis as well as how they featured in media narratives on the deadly nature of Ebola. In terms of blaming, prior work emphasizes the need to situate the analysis of the backlash against Africans within an understanding of blaming processes that emerged from the lack of order that characterized the initial response to the outbreak. The specific implications of blaming also need to be examined in ways that capture the experiences of both the stigmatized groups and the groups associated with the production of these stigmas.

Paying attention to prosocial responses should balance out the analysis of the overall response to the crisis. Accounts of the demonstration of agency provide a basis for investigating two related issues relevant to achieving this objective. The first relates to whether Africans in Dallas developed specific strategies to promote health functioning and to reduce their susceptibility to disease infection during the crisis. In other words, did African immigrants take specific actions to stop the spread of the Ebola virus within their communities? The second is whether these immigrants used broader demonstrations of agency to counter the narratives developed by the public to place the blame on them. Based on research on resilience, it is also important to extend the analysis beyond a focus on the initial disruption caused by the outbreak of the virus. Specifically, the question of how African immigrant groups targeted by stigma rebounded from these experiences throughout the course of the crisis further needs to be investigated. This process requires a broader articulation of how the actions of individuals and institutions provided a buffer that shielded communities from the brunt of the public backlash.

Weighing the evidence on this broad spectrum of responses allows us to move beyond simplistic notions of immigrant experiences during epidemics that are developed on the basis of the examination of negative responses only. While the experience of these negative responses is indisputable, the reality may be more complicated than it appears. For example, immigrants targeted by stigmas may also deploy stigmas against others in their communities. Similarly, the fear of Ebola need not be exclusive to local natives within the Dallas community but could also extend to immigrants themselves. These same types of complexities may characterize the prosocial responses observed during epidemics. Accordingly, effective demonstrations of agency among African immigrants may depend on the agency found among local residents who collaborated with them to mount a positive response to the crisis. These possibilities are what make the investigation of the implications of the Ebola crisis in Dallas intriguing. Among other things, they suggest that one set of responses does not necessarily preclude the experience of another, and that the actors involved in responding to these events are not neatly classifiable into mutually exclusive categories of heroes and villains.

A useful starting point for examining how these responses unfold is to locate them along the lines of Alcabes's (2009) proposed stages for understanding responses to epidemics. The first is the *physical event* observed at the start of the outbreak; the second, the *social crisis* created by this event; and the third, the *narrative* developed to understand what is being observed. Social responses to epidemics are observed in all three stages; however, Alcabes suggests that fear-based responses mainly emerge as part of the third stage. Significantly, however, previous accounts provide a strong case for adding a fourth stage, which is marked by the development of *counteractions*. This stage examines the responses used to combat the negative effects of the social crisis as well as the negative effects associated with the narratives of fear and blame.

Before examining these responses, though, it is important to describe the community context in which they were observed. A key dimension of this is the social organization of African communities in Dallas, and this is important for understanding the development of systems of vulnerability that made them susceptible to negative responses to the crisis. At the same time, these communities have developed unique social systems designed to help them withstand the consequences of emergencies. Whether these systems were able to withstand the backlash against the community during the outbreak is important and, as will be demonstrated shortly, a critical part of developing a comprehensive account of the social response to the crisis in Dallas.

3 Solidarity and Support among Africans in Dallas

Eight women in brightly colored clothes walk to the stage as congregants stand up to begin the Sunday service. They had arrived at the Ebenezer International Fellowship (EIF)* church earlier that morning, at its location about thirty minutes from downtown Dallas. While the EIF church is close to Dallas, its Sunday services are anything but American. As the women lead congregants in various songs of praise, a band plays tunes with a combination of African and Western instruments. African drums are played by a young man dressed in a Kente shirt, and not too far from him another person keeps the beat on an acoustic drum set. The rhythm is consistent and accompanied by melodies from a keyboard and a guitar played by musicians near the stage. Together, the band produces the lively music that breaks the morning silence. As congregants join in the morning singing, they dance to the beat, sometimes moving from their seats to find more space in the aisles. Near the wall by the women on the stage is a conspicuous row of flags that shows the countries whose nationals are represented in the church. The majority of them are from Africa. As such, there are flags for Kenya, South Africa, and Nigeria, along with flags of other countries in West Africa. However, there are two countries that have the most nationals represented in the church—Sierra Leone and Liberia. This is not a coincidence. Pastor Ken and his wife, the founders of the church, are nationals of these countries and have strong ties to the city's African community.

To a large extent, the EIF church represents the interconnected lives of African immigrants in Dallas. Although Pastor Ken was born in Liberia to

* A pseudonym is used here to preserve anonymity.

a Liberian mother and a Ghanaian father, he spent much of his adolescence in Sierra Leone before migrating to the United States. While in Sierra Leone, he completed his secondary education, played for a leading soccer team, and met his wife, with whom he now leads the church.

The EIF church also symbolizes the multidimensional nature of African immigrant institutions. As such, it is more than just a church, and this is not just because it eschews trappings of orthodoxy such as hymnals, choir robes, and organs. Apart from being a place of worship, it is also a place that caters to the diverse needs of its African members. It is the place where one goes to meet co-ethnics, socialize, and eat African food. Additionally, the church provides instrumental services that are essential for navigating the challenges of life as an immigrant. For example, it provides a community that has access to networks that new immigrants use in their search for employment. Members who need assistance with addressing immigration-related issues can also count on receiving advice from the church's lawyers and from long-term immigrants who also attend the church. Besides its focus on the spiritual needs of its members, therefore, the EIF is a multifaceted immigrant community. As a result, it plays a central role in the cultural, social, and emotional life of Africans in the city.

The EIF is not alone in the provision of these types of services. It is part of the larger array of African ethnic institutions whose functions are important for understanding the organization of social life in the community. Before the start of the Ebola crisis, Dallas witnessed a significant growth in African immigrant settlement, and this was followed by the development of systems of relationships, institutions, and alliances that were critical for advancing their social integration. At the same time, living in Dallas brought about several challenges for these new immigrants, who were not only Black but were living thousands of miles away from familiar systems of support in Africa. Unfazed by these challenges, they developed mechanisms to improve their access to resources and founded a number of ethnic organizations to promote various social and economic causes in their community. While the development of these systems is commendable, the African immigrant community is far from being self-sufficient. Indeed, the scale of African settlement and economic activity in Dallas has not expanded to the point where the community could be considered to be an ethnic enclave. This recognition is reserved for communities with large numbers of immigrants while also having high concentrations of ethnic firms that provide employment for co-ethnics (Portes and Jensen 1992). In this sense, the city's African community is less economically developed than those of immigrant groups such as the Chinese. Nevertheless, their social dynamics are important for developing a portrait of the contexts in which their response to the Ebola crisis was developed.

Constructing this portrait helps to fill the void created by the limited attention given to the social organization of African immigrant communities in the United States in general, or in Dallas in particular. With few exceptions (e.g., Moore 2013), previous studies give very little attention to why African immigrants settled in the city, the types of vulnerabilities they experience, and the main sources of their resilience. What explains the rapid growth of the African immigrant community in Dallas? How are these immigrants incorporated into systems of inequality that fall along fault lines associated with social tensions in the city? What types of re- sources do they have available that help to buffer them during periods of crisis? How do they leverage these resources to meet the needs of marginalized groups located in Dallas and those found in Africa?

As these questions are answered, it will become clear that African immigrant settlement in Dallas is a consequence of structural forces that operate both in their origin countries and within US society. With the establishment of these settlements, however, community life evolved in eclectic ways to help these immigrants establish firm roots in the city. Social structures were developed to expand their access to employment, mitigate immigration-related challenges, and navigate various types of crises. The foundational bases for the development of these structures are found in ethnic organizations. Over the years, these institutions have developed flexible systems for assisting immigrants bound by a common fate and by a set of shared social characteristics that could be traced to their origin countries. This bounded solidarity is a form of social capital found among groups whose members identify with one another under a specific set of circumstances and who, as a result of these bonds, provide altruistic support for members of their community (Portes 1998). Bounded solidarity is not based on a nebulous set of relationships. Instead, it is based on networks of family connections, friendships, and other common ties (Aguilera and Massey 2003; Portes and Sensenbrenner 1993). Working together with other mainstream American institutions decades before the Ebola epidemic, African ethnic institutions cultivated this source of social capital while also developing a track record of service to the less fortunate and responding to needs within their community.

The Allure of Dallas

Most scholars agree that the Hart-Celler Act, passed by the US Congress in 1965, laid the foundation for the recent growth in African immigration to the United States. Before then, emigration from regions other than Northern and Western Europe was restricted by various laws, including the National Origins Act of 1924. African immigration since 1965 has thus occurred as part of the largest wave of non-White immigrants arriving in the country since the end of slavery. Most immigrants arriving during this period settled in traditional gateway cities such as Chicago, New York, and Los Angeles. Two decades after the Hart-Cellar Act, however, the newly arrived immigrants included only modest numbers of Black immigrants from Africa and the Caribbean. Toward the end of the century, African immigration significantly increased, at a time when new emerging gateway cities were beginning to attract growing numbers of immigrants. Today, approximately one-third of the immigrant population of the United States lives in one of six such emerging gateway cities, including Houston, Riverside, the Dallas–Fort Worth (DFW) area, and Washington, DC (Singer 2015). In DFW itself, approximately one in six residents was an immigrant around the start of 2017 (Pappalardo 2017). More importantly, the area also hosted one of the largest concentrations of African immigrants living in the United States (Gambino et al. 2014).

US Census data on the arrival of immigrants in the DFW area indicate that this concentration of African immigrants is relatively recent. Accordingly, in the twenty-year period between 1950 and 1970, the proportion of residents who were African was consistently less than 1 percent (Ruggles et al. 2017). By the start of the 2014 Ebola crisis, this proportion had grown to approximately 6 percent of the total population. One-third of these immigrants were from West Africa, with the vast majority of them originating in Nigeria (71.1 percent). Compared to Nigeria, the shares of West Africans from Liberia (7.6 percent) and Sierra Leone (5.5 percent) were relatively small. However, this was enough for these two groups to account, respectively, for the third and fourth largest share of all West Africans in the area.

Why, then, are these immigrants migrating from Africa, and are there specific factors that make Dallas attractive to them? As previous studies have shown, the determinants of African migration to the United States are diverse; however, at least two of these determinants are among the most important. The first is the economic disparity between the United States and African countries, which fuels the drive to migrate and the chance at prosperity. Declining incomes, high unemployment, and the bleak economic outlook of many African countries all combine to make the decision to leave for greener pastures a rational choice for immigrants (Gordon 1998; Kent 2007). The effects of these influences are channeled through various pathways of immigration to the United States. For some, these pathways include enrolling in US higher education institutions, pursuing business opportunities, or migrating to join family members who are already in the country. Pursuing these dreams also involves traveling directly to the United States from their origin countries or through intermediary destination countries.

One example of the former is seen in the experience of François. He was born in the Democratic Republic of Congo but had no intention of migrating to the United States, even though he had dreams of living in the West. Realizing his options were limited because the DRC is a French-speaking country, he became more open to moving to the United States when he stumbled upon an opportunity to study abroad. As he put it, "I did not plan to come to the United States because of the French language. I said, 'Maybe I'll go to France or Belgium,' but the opportunity showed up for me to come here, so I came here, went to school here, and studied English first." Several years later, he earned a degree in the healthcare field, after which he started working for a state-level social service organization.

For other African immigrants, the journey to Dallas involved stepwise migrations to other countries, which were used as springboards for further migration to the United States. Among this group was Nancy, an immigrant from Sierra Leone who arrived in Texas more than thirty years ago. After leaving the country to train as a nurse in the United Kingdom in the mid-1970s, she assumed that she was at least going to spend some time there after her graduation, until she heard about the demand for nurses in

Texas. As a result, she left the United Kingdom after a few years and moved to Dallas, where she had a job offer from the hospital where she has worked ever since.

Like Nancy and François, other Africans who moved for economically related reasons have experienced some form of success, including Tayo, who arrived from Sierra Leone in the 1980s but now owns multiple businesses in the city; Brise, who left Cameroon for the United States several decades ago and settled in Dallas after earning his PhD; and Dr. Adu, an immigrant from Ghana who was also a successful medical doctor living in suburban Dallas. These people had another thing in common: they were part of an older cohort of immigrants who arrived in Dallas in the 1970s and 1980s, and who were now members of the city's professional class.

The second determinant of African migration to Dallas—refugee resettlement—mostly applied to more recent immigrants, especially those from Liberia and Sierra Leone. Both countries experienced interconnected civil wars around 1990, which led to significant levels of forced migration among their nationals. All this started in December 1989, when rebels from the National Patriotic Front of Liberia (NPFL), headed by Charles Taylor, invaded Liberia from neighboring Ivory Coast. The conflict continued for more than a decade and effectively ended with the exile of Taylor in 2003. At the start of the NPFL's rebellion, however, Taylor's forces received substantial help from a group led by Foday Sankoh, a former corporal in the Sierra Leonean army. Two years after the start of the Liberian civil war, Taylor returned the favor by helping Sankoh's rebel army start a civil war in neighboring Sierra Leone. Much of the recent increase in the West African population in Dallas is due to the resettlement of refugees from these countries because of these wars.

Such migrations speak to Texas's long history of participating in the resettlement of refugees from global conflicts. In fact, the state typically resettles some of the largest numbers of refugees in the country. Take, for example, what happened in 2015. In that year, the state hosted approximately 11 percent of all refugees arriving in the country, and this was the highest percentage observed across all US states (US Office of Refugee Resettlement 2016). Within Texas itself, the city of Dallas is a particularly attractive destination for refugee resettlement, and this is true for several reasons. It has a strong economy that offers refugees relatively easy access to low-skilled jobs, which helps them transition into the labor force. Its cost of living is comparatively lower than those of other major metropolitan areas, and, finally, the city has a well-developed public transit system that makes it easy for refuges to commute from their places of residence to their jobs. These factors not only explain why Dallas has become a useful landing spot for refugees from West Africa but also for refugees from countries such as Nepal, Afghanistan, and Iraq.

Accounts of the migration of African refugees to the city are as riveting as they are compelling. By the time they arrive in Dallas, many have experienced the tragedies, traumas, and changing fortunes associated with civil conflict. Take the case of Sam, a Liberian immigrant who now pastors a church Dallas. Back in Liberia, he was the proprietor of a successful foreign-exchange business, and the expansion of his clientele to include Lebanese merchants had all but guaranteed a future life of bliss. Then came the war, which increasingly put his life at risk. He was tempted to wait things out until the end of the hostilities; however, he fled the country as a last resort to save his life and start a new life elsewhere. By the time he decided to leave, he explained that

> everything [had] shut down; you couldn't go to school; you couldn't do business. I mean, we were literally in Liberia, and this was happening for more than three years. Your aspirations and dreams, and everything, were not moving in any way. Next, I started thinking, "Man, the next opportunity that comes, I'm out of here." I was one of those who knew the riches of our country. I never even wanted to travel, to leave Liberia, but when the civil war came, we had no choice. I mean, I was better off even in the crisis. . . . For each $100 bill that I converted into local currency I made a ten percent profit.

Leaving everything behind, Sam first attempted to migrate to neighboring Ivory Coast. To do this, though, he needed to avoid going through rebel-held territory because the NPFL was known for committing atrocities. Over the course of several weeks, he walked from his home in Monrovia, the capital city, to Lofa, close to the border with Ivory Coast—a distance of more than two hundred miles. Rejected by border guards who denied him entry into the country, he traveled to Guinea, and then to Sierra Leone, where he lived before resettling as a refugee in the United States in 1996.

Other Liberian refugees went through similar stepwise movements before their arrival in Dallas. Paul, like Sam, was also on a path to success
before his dreams were interrupted by the outbreak of hostilities. Seated in
the convenience store he now owns in Dallas, he gave the following recollection of his flight from conflict to the United States:

> I was at the university when the war began, and in 1989, we all had to leave the
> capital, leave the country. And then from there, I made my way over to Ivory
> Coast, and I was in Ivory Coast as a refugee for two and a half years. For a while
> in Ivory Coast, I was blessed and I got a job with the United Nations. I worked
> as an agricultural coordinator for the Liberian refugees. While serving in that
> position, I created a lot of jobs, let me say, created a lot of farms, and most of
> my farms were supplying the refugees in Danané. It was while I was in Ivory
> Coast that I got to meet some friends who informed me about the opportunity
> to travel to the US as a refugee.

What makes these flights from conflict particularly interesting is their
role in helping us understand how Louise Troh left Liberia for the United
States, as well as the circumstances in which she first met Thomas Duncan. As fighting between warring factions increased, Troh feared that she
was about to face a similar fate as her family members who died earlier in
the conflict. Her three siblings were killed during the fighting, and her aunt
died after soldiers burned her house down while she was still inside (Troh
2015). Like many Liberians, the first safe haven she sought was in neighboring Ivory Coast. Traveling from Liberia on foot, she often slept in the
forest, ate wild fruit, and drank water from creeks until she arrived at a
refugee camp in Danané, Ivory Coast (Troh 2015). It was while living in
the camp that she met Thomas Duncan, who was also there as a refugee at
the time, and started a romantic relationship with him. This relationship
was interrupted, however, after Louise was selected for the US Refugee
Resettlement Program. Unfortunately, Thomas was not. Consequently, she
left Ivory Coast for Dallas in 1998, where she lived until her reunification
with Thomas when he arrived in 2014.

Race, Class, and Social Vulnerability

Partly because of the diverse circumstances under which they arrive in
Dallas, African immigrants are exposed to a number of vulnerabilities that

put them at risk of negative social outcomes. Refugee groups, for example, have a history of trauma that can negatively affect social integration into their communities (Ellis et al. 2008). They also usually have high levels of food insecurity and low levels of English proficiency, and face a number of obstacles to their educational success (Darboe 2003; Hadley et al. 2007; McBrien 2005). Regardless of refugee status, however, all African immigrants face vulnerabilities associated with their race. Like other Black immigrants in the United States, their social incorporation occurs in a context that has historically been stratified by race (Krieger et al. 2011; Read and Emerson 2005). As such, their phenotypical characteristics make them targets of racism and prejudice more so than the respective characteristics of other immigrants. Several studies have thus provided evidence showing that Africans in Dallas report more personal experiences with prejudice or discrimination in their daily interactions compared to Hispanic or Asian immigrants. Specifically, they describe encounters Africans have with Americans who mock their accents, show that they are underpaid compared to similarly qualified coworkers, and document other direct experiences they have with racism and prejudice (Brettell 2011; Cordell and Griego 2005; Moore 2013). These reports were no different from accounts collected from current residents in the city. The most notable examples of these are an account of an interaction with a local resident who claimed an African immigrant with an accent reminded her of Tarzan and a conversation between an African immigrant and his coworker about whether Africans actually lived in houses.

Added to these are vulnerabilities created by the social tensions that accompanied the growth of the immigrant population in Dallas. While most residents in the city are perceived as being tolerant to new immigrants, some communities occasionally express strong opposition to the presence of these groups. In 2006, for example, Farmers Branch, a small town in the suburbs of Dallas, enacted a series of ordinances to restrict access to housing among immigrants thought to be undocumented and required managers to document the legal status of their tenants (Brettell and Nibbs 2010). Although the ordinance was ultimately struck down, it was proposed at the end of a thirty-year period that saw a fortyfold increase in the town's Hispanic population (Brettell and Nibbs 2010). Within Dallas itself, many residents have more accommodating views of immigrants, as reflected in their explicit shows of support for immigrants during rallies to promote immigration reform (Kreindler 2010). Nevertheless, national anti-immigration groups have a major presence in the city, and this muddles the social environment in which the integration of African immigrants occurs.

Another source of vulnerability among these immigrants is associated with their high levels of class stratification. Because of differences in their determinants of migration, access to opportunity, and years of US residence, African residents in the city have a highly bifurcated class structure. Long-term residents are part of a distinctive middle class, which includes immigrants who arrived as late as the 1980s and refugees who arrived in the 1990s. Many of these immigrants have experienced successful economic integration, secured high-paying jobs, and established a connection to larger social networks in the city. As they became successful, they also moved out to better neighborhoods in areas such as Garland, Euless, Hurst, and Irving. Consequently, they have joined a growing number of highly successful immigrant groups in the area, including highly skilled immigrants from India who work at local universities, the nuclear plant at Comanche Peak, and companies such as Texas Instruments (Brettell 2005). These middle-class Africans also have high levels of human capital—they have high levels of English proficiency, are more educated than some local natives, and in some cases arrived in the United States as skilled workers recruited by American employers (Cordell and Griego 2005).

At the other end of the class spectrum are working-class Africans who have not yet been able to achieve the American Dream. They include refugees from Somalia, Sudan, and Liberia, as well as long-term US residents whose social mobility is constrained by their limited levels of human capital. This group also includes college-educated immigrants who cannot use their credentials earned in Africa in the US labor market and as a result have opted to pursue other ventures, such as hair-braiding. More importantly, this lower class of Africans is among the most socially vulnerable and economically disadvantaged in the city. They work in low-skilled jobs, have poor English-speaking skills, and live in the poorest neighborhoods in the city. One such neighborhood is Vickery Meadow, where Louise Troh lived in 2014 and which was at the center of the Ebola crisis that gripped the city of Dallas.

Vickery Meadow and the Socially Disadvantaged

The neighborhood now referred to as Vickery Meadow was a thriving farming community before it was annexed by the city of Dallas in 1945 (Jacobson 1996). Shortly thereafter, investors started pouring in and developed the area into a fashionable residential district that was supposed to attract young working couples (*Dallas Morning News* 2000). Its first housing options were complexes with one-bedroom apartments of about five hundred square feet (Jacobson 1996). When its first residents started to arrive in the early 1970s, Vickery Meadow had been developed into a fashionable neighborhood with swimming pools and a prominent night-life that added to its social scene (Jacobson 1996). But the fortunes of the neighborhood changed with the downturn in the real estate market in the late 1980s. As its young residents departed, thousands of apartments and condominiums became vacant, and were quickly converted into low-income rental units (Jacobson 2006).

The new residents of these units included Hispanic immigrants in search of affordable housing and poor families of other racial minority groups (Jacobson 1996). As the number of low-income renters increased, the neighborhood also became known for its high population density. Its core residential area hosted approximately 41,000 people who lived in a space of less than three square miles (Young 2006). As if this was not enough, the community experienced a decline in municipal investment as well as an inadequate provision of social services, which accelerated its transformation from a dynamic community into one synonymous with blight.

It did not take long for Vickery Meadow to develop a reputation as a place people should avoid (Young 2006). Crime rates had increased to among the highest in the city. In one ten-month period, for example, more than two hundred home break-ins were reported in the neighborhood's approximately three-mile radius (Picket 2012). Indeed, some residents referred to Vickery Meadow as the crime capital of Dallas. Criminal activities occurred in plain sight, including those of prostitutes and drug dealers, who frequently plied their trade on neighborhood streets (*Dallas Morning News* 2000; Young 2006). At sunrise, these prostitutes walked the streets as parents walked their children to school buses (Jacobson 2006). At night, violent crimes increased to the point that apartment complexes constructed electronic or high concrete fences to provide residents with some sense of security. To many locals, these measures were understandable. At one point, the number of convicts in the neighborhood became so high that the government opened an adult probation office there to provide supervision for those doing community service (*Dallas Morning News* 2000).

By the time Louise Troh arrived at Vickery Meadow, the neighborhood had become a local source of stigma. Its residents were seen as troublemakers living in a community described as a fire that feeds on itself and a place were victims and criminals lived together (*Dallas Morning News* 2000). Living in Vickery Meadow meant living in hopelessness, in poverty, and in a place where few people wanted to go. As one commentator described the neighborhood, it was a place once considered an Eden for singles that had been transformed into a paradise lost (Young 2006). Yet, the ultimate marker of the stigmatization of the neighborhood was still to come. It was the local use of the term "Meadow Ghetto" to describe the community, and the term emphasized its ghetto status as well as its association with substandard housing, poverty, and crime (Zethraus 1994).

At the turn of the century, new efforts were started to invest in the neighborhood's dilapidated infrastructure and to improve its overall image. Apartment buildings were spruced up, and the community was connected to a light rail station built in the Park Lane area as part of a $400 million public transit project (Jacobson 2006). The most rundown apartments were demolished to make way for the construction of new schools. Activists, churches, and community organizations also became more involved. They helped develop a crime watch group, an after-school program, and other programs that provided free summer lunches and recreational activities for children in the neighborhood (Zethraus 1994). However, some of the old problems with prostitution remained, even though crime rates significantly declined (Jacobson 2006). To many observers, however, the stigma of the neighborhood remained (*Dallas Morning News* 2000). The negative image of Vickery Meadow remained ingrained in their minds despite the improvement in living conditions and access to services.

Today, the neighborhood hosts one of the most racially diverse communities in Dallas. This diversity is typically on display during routine activities such as the arrival of school buses at the end of the school day.

On a recent summer afternoon, for example, the buses stopped adjacent to the wall of a building covered with posters advertising free English classes and other social services available to refugee families in the area. As the children exited the buses, they revealed notable markers of the racial and ethnic composition of the neighborhood. Backpack-carrying girls wearing hijabs walked to the sidewalk with their Asian and Hispanic friends. Not too far behind were Black kids who walked up to adults wearing traditional African clothing who had been waiting near the curb to pick them up. The community has become so diverse that it is now referred to as the United Nations. Its residents come from countries such as Bosnia, Sudan, Burundi, Afghanistan, and more recently from Iraq. A few others are members of older refugee groups, such as those from Liberia, who choose to remain in the community because of its proximity to their places of employment or because of their lack of resources to move to the wealthy suburbs.

Because of its abundance of low-income housing, easy access to public transportation, and proximity to low-skill jobs, the neighborhood has also become the most attractive option for housing-resettled refugees in Dallas. For resettlement agencies in the city, the low cost of living in Vickery Meadow allows them to stretch the fix amount of funding they receive from the US government to cover the provision of services to refugees. Few neighborhoods in the city have apartment complexes willing to accept the fix amount of rental payments for refugees that these agencies are allowed to make. Moreover, because the rental support provided to refugees lasts for less than a year, remaining in the neighborhood allows them to continue to live near institutions such as schools and places of employment, which are critical for advancing their incorporation into society. For many low-income Africans, these advantages are hard to ignore.

Community Institutions and African Immigrant Life

As a result of these variations in place of residence, social class, and life circumstances, community life among African immigrants is organized to provide opportunities for forming alliances that are instrumental for ameliorating their challenges. The most important sources of these opportunities are found in immigrant organizations, that is, the wide range of religious, cultural, and humanitarian organizations founded by Africans in the city. The resources they provide are supplemented by those provided by mainstream institutions that connect them to wider social networks in Dallas. Collectively, African immigrant institutions help residents cope with racial stereotypes, adapt to their new environment, and navigate the dynamics of social disadvantage in their communities (Takougang and Tidjani 2009).

Before examining the significance of specific immigrant institutions, however, it is important to identify several broad characteristics that are important for understanding how these institutions adapt to serve the needs of their members. One of these attributes is immigrant institutions' dynamic patterns of membership. Affiliation with specific organizations is the outcome of individual assessments of the extent to which the available options can fulfill their practical needs. Therefore, becoming a member of the EIF church does not preclude membership to other specialized organizations that provide other types of resources. These include cultural associations, alumni organizations of leading schools in Africa, or human services organizations. The flexible strategies used for raising and distributing resources by each of these organizations can be leveraged in ways that allow immigrants to comprehensively respond to crises.

Related to these dynamic patterns of membership is the ability of these organizations to adapt to the needs of their members by performing a diversity of functions. Three of these are among the most important. The first is the provision of cultural functions that attempt to replicate various aspects of community life in Africa. These functions are critical for two reasons: (1) they help African immigrants stay connected with the cultures of their origin countries, and (2) they help them distinguish themselves from local residents in a way that reinforces their pride in their ethnicity (Schrover and Vermeulen 2005).

A second function of these organizations is the promotion of stronger connections between African immigrants and mainstream institutions in the city. Accordingly, they provide mechanisms that allow members to access social capital from a wider network of institutions and to build bridges with local citizens that are essential for addressing common interests. In this sense, these immigrant institutions facilitate the social integration of Africans into the community. The most common strategies used to meet these goals include the promotion of responsible citizenship, local political participation, and service to the community. By building bridges with other local citizens, African immigrant organizations create pathways for the transmission of ideas and resources between themselves and natives that are mutually beneficial.

The third function is to foster ties between the African immigrant community in Dallas and various countries in Africa. These connections facilitate the extension of immigrants' social, economic, and political influence across international space and allow them to function as transnational subjects. Such transnational connections allow African immigrants, for example, to use resources located in the United States to fund political activities or participate in altruist endeavors such as economic development in poor African communities.

Beyond the diversity of their functions, these immigrant institutions are also characterized by their tendency to be aligned with demographic and social differences within the African immigrant population. Apart from the fact that these immigrants have diverse national origins, they also have notable ethnic differences that exist within national groups. This diversity has important implications for the organization of African immigrant institutions. On the one hand, it leads to the proliferation of immigrant-led institutions as each group tries to create a space for its members to develop a sense of belonging. On the other hand, it can constrain the development of pan-national or pan-African organizations, which help African immigrants speak with one voice.

Finally, African immigrant institutions are characterized by their high levels of operational fluidity, that is, their tendency to extend their operations beyond the central scope of their functions. While cultural associations typically focus on the preservation of the premigration customs and traditions of ethnic groups, they occasionally extend their reach to the performance of humanitarian and social functions. Similarly, religious organizations do not just focus on the provision of spiritual support but also frequently support social events such as picnics designed with the goal of improving social bonds within the community. This operational fluidity is as much of a reflection of the diverse needs found in the community as it is a reflection of community members' ability to leverage resources.

Having developed a general sense of the main attributes of immigrant organizations serving Africans in Dallas, we can now examine their interconnected influence on how these organizations serve their members as well as how these services are deployed during times of need. The examination focuses on two broad types of organizations: those based on social identities (i.e., ethnic/cultural and national identities) and those that focus on providing specialized functions (i.e., churches and human services organizations).*

Serving Immigrants and Responding to Their Needs

Naming ceremonies are elaborate events used for celebrating the birth of children among many African ethnic groups. As such, the birth of a child among Mandingo immigrants, who are from West Africa, provides a unique opportunity to celebrate the cultural practices of the group. One such event was a two-day celebration in Dallas that started with a traditional meet-and-greet ceremony at the house of the local Mandingo chief. Dressed in their colorful African attire, the guests arrived from various places in Texas as well as from states including Illinois, New Jersey, and Wisconsin. Upon entry into the house, the distinct seating patterns were impossible to miss.† Women and men sat in separate sections of the living room, respectively forming circles around several communal food trays. The menu included jollof rice, meat stews, and different types of vegetables.

After dinner, the formal part of the ceremony commenced and was conducted almost entirely in the Mandingo language. As part of the ceremony, each guest was presented to the chief by the chief's attendant and was allowed to give a brief speech thanking the chief for providing care for the new parents during the pregnancy. After about an hour, the chief gave brief remarks, indicating the end of the formal ceremony. Almost immediately thereafter, a traditional praise singer began to sing in melodious tones that could be heard even by those outside the house. She started by

---

* This distinction is used for analytical simplicity. In reality, some immigrant organizations are established on the basis of social identities while also performing specialized functions.

† I was invited to the meeting by one of the leaders of a Mandingo cultural group in the city. Since I do not understand Mandingo, my host served as an interpreter for much of the meeting.

rendering extravagant praises to the chief,* after which she ad-libbed songs about each guest, celebrating the exploits of their ancestors, whom she was able to identify based on their last names.

Cultural organizations such as those formed by the Mandingos are organizations that strictly serve members who identify with an ethnic group. They attract a more consistent following compared to national-level organizations, because most Africans place a higher significance on their ethnic identity than on their national identity (Takougang and Tidjani 2009). This practice has several advantages. In particular, it allows cultural groups to leverage the high level of commitment of its members to raise funds to undertake projects that benefit their community. Moreover, it provides a special place of belonging for immigrants with a shared set of cultural values.

Of the more than 1,600 ethnic communities and international-themed organizations in the DFW area, there are at least sixty that serve the African immigrant community (Sanchez and Weiss-Armuch 2003). Most of these organizations are found among larger nativity groups, such as Ethiopians and Nigerians. These groups are also among the most culturally diverse. Based on ethnicity, for example, Nigerian immigrants could choose to become a member of organizations that exclusively serve Yorubas or Igbos, or they could become members of any of the forty-five Nigerian cultural organizations found in the community (Sanchez and Weiss-Armuch 2003). Among Liberians, Guineans, and Sierra Leoneans, ethnic configurations are significantly less diverse. Nevertheless, these immigrants can choose to belong to cultural groups that serve Mandingos, Fullahs, Krios, Mendes, or the other major ethnic groups from their country represented in the city.

While each group's central objective is to preserve cultural traditions practiced in Africa, they frequently pursue other secondary objectives. Most

* The praise singer started her routine by singing the praises of the chief. My host provided an interpretation of the words of this first song: "A chief is not someone who is extraordinary. There is a reason why you have a title of a chief because it is a very outstanding position. You are a man of honor; you are a man of dignity." Everyone was in a jubilant mood and cheering while she sang. They were more jubilant while she sang praises to the chief, and as she did so, the men surrounding the chief raised his hands as they danced with him.

of them have programs designed to raise funds among their members to support less fortunate co-ethnics within the city or in Africa. Each year, for example, the Krio organization in Dallas conducts a fund-raising event to support scholarships for Krio students in Sierra Leone. Occasionally, they also raise funds for special programs such as one that refurbished a clinic in a poor community in the country. Like the Krios, Mandingo immigrants in the city have long-standing traditions associated with raising funds for projects in Liberia. One of them is an annual event during which members seek donations of medicine and medical equipment from hospitals in the Dallas area, which are then collected and shipped to Liberia.

Within the city, the other secondary objectives of cultural organizations are almost exclusively designed with the goal of promoting the social and economic welfare of their members. One of the best examples of this is the informal job referral services found among the Mandingos. New Mandingo immigrants who are unemployed are usually referred to job networks in the transportation industry, since this is where a large number of Mandingos are employed. In fact, there is an emerging Mandingo ethnic niche in the industry, which is reflected in the large number of co-ethnics who drive taxicabs and airport shuttles in the city of Dallas. Another secondary objective of cultural organizations is to mitigate the consequences of tragedy in the community. Ethiopian immigrants, for example, founded a cultural association organized around the traditional practice of *edir* (i.e., burial society), which provides financial assistance to members during times of bereavement. The process requires members to make monthly financial contributions to the association, which are pooled into a general fund that is used to cover funeral expenses for members and their families.

Ethnic differences among Africans in the community are nevertheless deemphasized in favor of broader displays of unity during periods of tragedy. Evidence of this was observed during the death of a newly arrived Eritrean immigrant in Dallas. The immigrant had never before seen a freeway, and he died as he attempted to cross it (Meyers 2008). Following this incident, there was a large show of unity among Africans in the city as well as a commitment to build alliances among local ethnic groups (Meyers 2008). Similar collective responses have been observed among African immigrants elsewhere in the United States. Among the most notable was the death of Ahmed Diallo, an immigrant from Guinea, who was shot forty-one times in a case of police brutality in New York. In what was a massive show of support following the death of Diallo, hundreds of Africans turned out to protest against the police in the city (Hule 1999).

Although collaborative efforts such as these are rare among African immigrants, they can still be observed on a smaller scale within national-origin immigrant organizations. Community members use these organizations as forums for advancing the collective interests of nativity groups, and this objective is typically pursued by coordinating the activities of the ethnic organizations respectively serving these groups. Beyond these functions, national-origin associations provide an added buffer to protect members who are faced with emergencies. Indeed, the origins of one such organization, the Council of Liberian Associations (CLA),* is specifically tied to an emergency that occurred in the recent past. Slightly more than three decades ago, a Liberian resident died in the city, and because he did not have life insurance, his family was unable to afford the cost of his funeral. Prominent Liberian immigrants then stepped in to organize a campaign that successfully raised funds to meet the needs of the family. To prevent the reoccurrence of such unfortunate circumstances, they decided to form the CLA, with the initial goal of providing a system of mutual assistance to address similar needs in the future. Today, national-level organizations such as the CLA, the Ivorian Community Association, and the Organization of Sierra Leoneans in Texas mainly focus on common issues of concern related to their respective countries of origin. Accordingly, they bring together immigrants from their countries to celebrate national holidays and occasionally lobby governments in their homelands to promote various social causes.

Service to Immigrants in Church and Human Services Organizations

Other African immigrant organizations are based not so much on ethnic or national identities but on the provision of specialized types of services. Arguably the most important of these found in the African immigrant

---

* As mentioned earlier, these organizations are identified using pseudonyms. It is also important to note that African nationalities represented among immigrants in Dallas do not have such organizations.

community are church organizations. Christianity, Islam, and animism are the three major religions practiced in Africa, with Christianity experiencing one of the most rapid rates of growth on the continent in recent decades (PEW Forum 2010). Partly because of this growth, there has also been a tremendous increase in the number of African immigrant churches in US cities since the 1980s.* Like other local churches, African churches in Dallas primarily exist to meet the spiritual needs of their members. These needs are met in a uniquely African way, with worship services tapping into norms, mores, and symbols associated with traditional African life.

Listening to Sam describe why he started a Liberian church in Dallas helps to shed light on how these factors influence his goal of providing religious services to co-ethnics in the city. Drawing from his own roots in Liberia, he explained the importance of having a church experience that reminded his congregants of home. Many of the songs are traditional songs that are sung in churches in Liberia. In this way, the church experience culturally resonates with the members of Sam's church and adds a unique dimension to their worship experience that is missing from other churches in the city. As Sam further explained, another advantage of having a Liberian church is that it puts congregants in contact with a pastor with whom they can identify. In other words, Sam was someone familiar with the anxieties of dealing with the immigration system, separation from family members back home, and experiences of marginalization, prejudice, and rejection. As such, his congregants could relate more closely with him than they could with other pastors in the city.

Owing to their marginalization, African immigrant churches have evolved in ways that are similar to that observed in the early origins of the African American church. At that time, slave owners prohibited the development of such institutions out of fear that they would provide a cover for planning rebellions (Maffly-Kipp 2001). As a result, the slaves developed secret hush harbors as places of worship, where they combined African songs with their beliefs in Christianity (Maffly-Kipp 2001; Moore 1991). Like contemporary African immigrant churches, these institutions served as places where African traditions could be incorporated into the worship

---

* In New York alone, approximately 110 new African immigrant churches were established between 1980 and 2004 (Chan 2004).

experience, and they also served as places of refuge that for a brief moment could shield members from the prejudices encountered in everyday life (Maffly-Kipp 2001; Moore 1991).

This connection between the African immigrant churches and the African American church was not lost on Sam. Indeed, he embraced it. He observed that, like the latter, the former allows its members to develop a sense of worth, which is usually lacking in their daily interactions in the city. Expanding this line of thought, he observed the following: "It's almost like [during] slavery. During slavery, the only place where the Black man had a voice was in the church; think about it. And that's why [our] churches always have a lot of problems because everybody wants to talk. At their place of work, they can't talk. They're not decision makers. They say, 'Yes, sir,' all day long, 'Yes sir, yes sir, yes ma'am.' The church is the only place where they can come and have a voice."

Apart from this, African churches provide a place where members receive inspirational messages that encourage them to face the challenges of life as immigrants. At the EIF church, the vibrant singing and dancing is usually followed by an uplifting sermon from Pastor Ken, a charismatic and skilled orator. In one sermon, for example, he used the popular biblical story of David and Goliath to develop an underdog metaphor, which he then used to encourage his members to persevere so that they may one day achieve the American Dream.

Integrated into the programs of many of these churches, however, is the provision of various types of nonspiritual services. Accordingly, in Pastor Ken's view, the need to attend to the nonspiritual needs of his parishioners was as much a part of his calling as was the delivery of spiritual direction. He did not see this approach as contradictory; instead, he saw it as complementary. In his view, it was a sort of full-service approach that he needed to embrace in order to serve the needs of Africans. He described it as follows:

> Whilst it is true that every church is called to preach spirituality, I was called to go beyond spirituality and include the other needs of man because mankind is a three-part being. We are a spirit, we have a soul, and we live in a body, and so my church is very holistic like that. We have an immigration lawyer; we have a civil lawyer; we have everything. Everything that relates to my people, I reach

out and find a partner that I can work with, because it's not just about preaching John 3:16 and after they leave the doors of the church, then that's it, but it's about following them, so we do a lot.

By "a lot," he is referring to providing immigration advice to members as well as informal job referrals. The kitchen on the church's premises allows members to serve meals during wedding receptions and the informal gatherings that frequently occur at the end of Sunday services. These times of fellowship are important because they allow members to socialize in what the pastor referred to as an "African way." In other words, his congregants are permitted to socialize as they eat free African meals, which include palm butter stew or potato greens and usually rice.

Because African immigrant churches are close-knit communities, they also serve as a first stop for crisis control for immigrants facing various types of emergencies. For example, the EIF church provides resources for bailing out youth charged with committing petty crimes in the city. Additionally, because the pastor is a trained counselor, he regularly offers counseling for troubled youth, bereaved members, and members dealing with marital problems. At Unity Fellowship, another church founded by Liberians, the process of responding to emergencies is even more structured. The church maintains a database containing information on members with immediate needs, which is also used to allocate resources to families during periods of crisis. Furthermore, when a congregant loses a family member in Africa, the church not only helps by providing material support to the bereaved but also sends text messages to all parishioners informing them of the bereavement and encouraging them to call the bereaved to express their condolences.

Outside church organizations, Africans in Dallas can also tap into the resource offered by human services organizations in the city. Some of these organizations, such as the International Rescue Committee, the Catholic Charities of Dallas, and the Refugee Services of Texas, provide the first contact with US institutions for African refugees from war-affected countries. However, the growing refugee presence in Dallas has resulted in two other transformations in the landscape of humanitarian organizations in the city. The first is the establishment of African-led organizations that also provide services to refugees and other immigrants in the city. The second is the growth of similar African-led organizations that focus on the delivery of relief services to disadvantaged populations in Africa. Together, these transformations represent manifestations of the recent emergence of African organizations exclusively dedicated to serving those in need. Leaders of these organizations sometimes include former refugees, who draw from their own experiences to establish organizations that provide social services locally and internationally.

Life as a refugee from Liberia was therefore what inspired Paul to start a small humanitarian organization called the African Refugee Service Agency (ARSA). While receiving assistance from the US government in the early years after his arrival, he also volunteered at the church he attended to help other refugees who were resettling in the city. This volunteer position required him to work in the church's food pantry and to assist in the distribution of clothing, furniture, and other essentials needed to start life in the United States. His desire to provide similar services to Africans was what led him to establish the ARSA, which had the initial goal of serving the needs of new Liberian refugees in the city.

Other established immigrants start new organizations by capitalizing on the high demand for social services among new African immigrants in order to provide other types of services. One example of this was François, who realized the need to leverage the high demand for his French–English bilingual skills from immigrant-serving institutions. It started with calls he received from hospitals looking for someone to provide language translation services for immigrants from his native Congo. While working as a translator, he identified a wider range of social services needed by these newly arriving immigrants. Therefore, he used his training in public health, as well as his connections in the health field, to start an organization that provided a six-month training program for certified nursing assistants who could be immediately employed after graduation.

African immigrant–led human services organizations occasionally extend their aid outside US borders to engage in various types of transnational relief operations. These ventures usually stem from a desire to advance philanthropic endeavors in their origin countries using financial and social capital acquired from the West (Portes 2009). Such displays of transnational philanthropy contradict the notion that the loss of human capital from developing countries through migration represents a net loss to the continent (Portes 2009). Improvements in technology now allow immigrants to give back by using the rapid transfer of information on humanitarian needs abroad to develop philanthropic interventions to help the poor (De Haas 2010).

Two types of human services institution participate in the transnational activities of Africans in Dallas. The first are sole proprietorships driven by the efforts of individuals altruistically responding to the needs of poor Africans. They are usually founded by immigrants with an entrepreneurial spirit who capitalized on what they perceived to be the failure of conventional humanitarian organizations to respond to disadvantaged populations on the continent. Because of their low start-up costs, many of these organizations are run by their founders, and they rely on whatever help they can get from people sympathetic to their causes.

Paul's organization became one such sole proprietorship after he decided to expand the focus of ARSA to include service not only to local refugees but to war-affected communities in Liberia. However, the transnational arm of his organization was simply based on periodic trips to Liberia to take relief supplies collected from members of his Dallas network. In Liberia, his work further benefited from his connection to a small network of stakeholders who helped to distribute supplies after they arrived in the country. He described how the process worked with regard to a trip he took to the country in 2007:

> I carried a lot of back-to-school supplies and other things, okay. Stationery and school books, materials for school, chairs, and children's clothes, women's clothes—everything—and when I went in 2007 I worked along with [an international development agency]. My cousin was one of the directors. He gave me one of their trucks, then we began to unload the container [and] take the clothes to an orphanage on the Kakata Highway near Monrovia and even to churches like Calvary Baptist Church on Tubman Boulevard. I gave clothes out to them, and to groups in another district in Nimba called Dompa. The people received a lot of clothes. I had big, fat bundles of clothes, and I gave them to the people.

Josiah, who arrived in Dallas from Sierra Leone in the mid-1990s, ran a similar individually operated venture, and his motivation to start his organization was to help people whose limbs had been amputated during the country's civil war. Responding to media coverage of the war after he arrived in the United States, he asked members of his church for donations of used items he could send home to help victims of the war. During the process of accepting donations of used clothes, shoes, and other items, he formed a humanitarian organization to help the less fortunate in Sierra Leone and, later, in countries such as Haiti.

Many other immigrants are further engaged in informal ventures that seek to provide relief supplies or promote economic development in their countries of origin. Some of them make periodic trips back home to fund projects, help during emergencies, and provide humanitarian aid to their communities. In this way, they remain in touch with Africa in ways that allow them to participate in two worlds located across international space.

A second type of such transnational activity involves those tied to the activities of more formal ethnic organizations. A loose form of such activities are those associated with the secondary functions of these organizations, including periodic fund-raising activities with the goal of supporting education or providing basic social infrastructure in Africa. A more structured form of such activities is found in organizations that conduct more systematic transnational activities between Dallas and Africa. Some of these are tied to groups that conduct annual medical missions trips to the region, while others involve partnerships with local organizations such as church groups that conduct similar trips.

For example, several years after Nancy came to the United States from Sierra Leone in the 1970s, she became a member of a group that conducted periodic medical missions trips to her homeland. This group was an organization made up of healthcare professionals that periodically traveled to Sierra Leone to provide services to the sick. As a nurse, she thought this was the least she could do to help the country recover from its civil war since she had been in the United States before the start of the conflict. As she explained, "After the war in Sierra Leone, I really had something tugging at my heart and letting me know that I needed to do something—my own contribution to healthcare in Sierra Leone. So I started going on missions trips, and my first trip actually was nonmedical—right after the war, which was in 2000, March of 2000, and then in 2002, I went on my first medical mission with a Nigerian doctor and his group who were going to Sierra Leone after the war, and I got hooked." This was the start of a new engagement with her country that helped her develop a connection with poor communities. Moreover, the periodic visits were essential for developing connections with healthcare institutions in the country that were later affected by the Ebola crisis.

By and large, therefore, the evidence on the operations of African ethnic organizations in the Dallas area indicates that there were at least two types of practices central to their operations before the start of the epidemic. The first was the tradition of meeting the cultural, social, and economic needs of co-ethnics. This was done both locally and in their extended communities in their home countries. The second was the development of systems of collecting resources and other types of material support that helped them meet their primary and secondary objectives. Similar practices have been found among other immigrants in the United States, including those from Eastern Europe, the Philippines, and other Southeast Asian countries (Majka and Mullan 2002; Opiniano 2005). However, the examination of such operations among Africans in Dallas highlights a key feature of the social organization of their communities before the start of the Ebola crisis; that is, they had ways of mitigating various types of social challenges. Additionally, they had functional systems for responding to the needs of their members that underscored their ability to be resilient.

Crisis, Survival, and Resilience in African Immigrant Communities

Over time, life for African immigrants in Dallas evolved in ways that exposed them to a number of issues that provided obstacles to their integration into the community. These issues ranged from the need to navigate life as newcomers in the city to complex issues that negatively affected their welfare. There were at least three complex challenges that needed to be addressed. The first was associated with their bifurcated class structure and the disadvantage of lower class status. The second was their routine exposure to marginalization on the basis of their race. The third was related to their experiences of unfortunate events such as bereavement, unemployment, and unforeseen economic crises. In addition to these were more general concerns, such as the initial isolation that comes with living away from their communities in Africa.

Decades before the Ebola crisis in the city, however, the process of responding to these issues had resulted in the development of several types of systems that helped African immigrants resiliently respond in the face of crisis. The first was a system of bounded solidarity (Portes 1998). Common bonds formed on the basis of a shared fate and reinforced by shared social attributes were used to cultivate local sources of social capital to advance the welfare of co-ethnics. Indeed, the diverse range of ethnic institutions in the community provided many opportunities for developing connections to such systems of support. Outside these institutions, however, there were informal arrangements used to support those in need based on larger bonds of shared identity, such as those related to national origins. For instance, at the EIF church unemployed nonmembers were still provided with access to informal job referral services by members who were socially connected to employers in the city.

Notwithstanding these displays of solidarity, common bonds among African immigrants are sometimes at risk of being weakened by the influence of larger social forces. Long-held political grievances and ethnic tensions originating in Africa can create the potential for strained relations among immigrants from different groups from the same countries. Ethnic loyalties can further negatively influence attendance at social events and undermine the process of developing consensus on national issues affecting the country. Nevertheless, these competing interests are overlooked during crises that have threatened the welfare of the community.

Another strategy used for developing resilient responses was the cultivation of various mechanisms for managing such crises. Adapting to life in Dallas has required African immigrants to establish direct ways of responding to emergencies that are faced by co-ethnics. Out of these responses has emerged a series of specific strategies used during these periods. They include the development of systems that alert members of ethnic organizations to trigger a community response to bereavement, support systems to pay for funeral expenses, and mechanisms used for bailing out troubled youth who are arrested. Although the development of these strategies is important, it does not imply that the interventions themselves are perfect. Instead, it points to the existence of a willingness among African immigrants to provide material assistance to co-ethnics during emergencies. Additionally, it speaks to the presence of a system of coinsurance that helps to buffer members of the community during times of need.

At the same time, their ability to respond in times of crisis depends on their connection to broader social networks, which allow them to tap into resources from outside the African immigrant community. In part, this stems from the fact that ethnic institutions have established well-built partnerships with organizations in the city that assist them in their efforts to provide humanitarian services. Paul's organization was thus connected to a network of local church institutions, while Mandingo immigrants were connected to a network of local healthcare providers. In both cases, these connections existed long before the start of the Ebola crisis. Significantly, however, these connections understate the degree to which African immigrants are embedded within larger social networks within the city. As they experienced social mobility, longer-term African residents amassed social capital by establishing relationships with a wide range of public- and private-sector institutions. They served on school boards and on municipal councils; they worked at local banks and as higher education professionals. These connections gave them access to a broader set of resources— resources that could be used to provide them with services that they could not access on their own.

A final mechanism that African immigrants used to respond in times of crisis was their participation in transnational philanthropic work. Among other things, these activities were important because they involved the transfer of resources from the United States to various African countries. Their operational flexibility made it possible for ethnic organizations to participate in these activities and allowed them to gain experience with activities such as fund-raising and the development of relationships with organizations based in Africa. Furthermore, they had access to complementary resources in national-origin immigrant groups, which had contacts with governments in African countries, as well as to local stakeholders in Africa, which helped to advance their transnational activities.

Altogether, these mechanisms helped to increase the resilience of the African community in Dallas prior to the start of the Ebola crisis. Nevertheless, at no point in time had they been tested on a scale as significant as that ushered by the death of Thomas Duncan. Indeed, the community had never faced a crisis so significant that it put their lives at risk. It also never had to respond to a crisis while facing an unprecedented level of backlash from other city residents. In short, although African ethnic institutions had been effective in responding to various challenges in the past, there was no way of knowing whether they could handle an Ebola epidemic of such global significance. How they responded to this event is important for understanding how periods of acute vulnerability affect social life in immigrant communities. The first wave of this vulnerability was experienced at the start of the outbreak in West Africa, and the early responses of the community provide insights into how the social response to an epidemic unfolds.

4 Experiencing the Consequences of the Epidemic in West Africa

A decade after arriving in the United States, Bishop Charles Roberts became one of the first people to establish a church for Liberian immigrants in the Dallas area. This milestone was significant. It was achieved after he graduated from a Christian college, thereby fulfilling his original objective for migrating to the United States. A few years after starting his church, Roberts was appointed as the overseer of several Liberian churches in the city. But he was more than just a spiritual leader. In his more than thirty years of living in Dallas, he had developed a reputation as a respected elder whom many Liberian immigrants referred to as their grandfather. Beyond the United States, however, his influence was most felt in his native Liberia, where he continued to provide pastoral oversight to churches. Much of this took place on annual visits to the country, during which he also provided support to humanitarian organizations and checked in with the school he had established there.

In early 2014, Roberts took a break from this routine to visit Monrovia, Liberia, on a vacation. He was there with his family to celebrate the fact that James, his son, had just graduated from high school. Before leaving for Liberia, they read on Facebook that a deadly virus was spreading in Guinea. This was disturbing but not significant enough to warrant canceling their plans. The first couple days after arriving in Monrovia were exciting, especially for James, who had made frequent visits to the YMCA to socialize with his friends. A few days later, the first case of Ebola in Monrovia was confirmed. Five people were diagnosed with the virus, and this signaled the need for the Roberts family to be more vigilant. Shortly thereafter, James came down with a fever, and his dad tried to dismiss the possibility that he had contracted Ebola at the YMCA. However, the longer the fever lasted, the more Roberts's fears increased. James's symptoms were difficult to ignore, and they were becoming very similar to those observed at the onset of an Ebola infection. Fearing the worst, the bishop offered James some Tylenol and stayed up praying throughout the night. By the next morning, the fever was gone. It was a close call, but the Roberts family knew that some things had to change. James no longer visited the YMCA, while everyone else tried to avoid crowded areas. Fortunately for them, the plan worked. They remained uninfected for the remainder of their trip, and they returned to Dallas before the scale of the epidemic increased.

Like the Roberts family, many Africans in Dallas largely depend on social media to receive up-to-date information about what is going on at home. However, around the start of the epidemic, these sources provided limited information on the threat of the outbreak occurring in Guinea, making assessment difficult. Everyone knew that life back in Africa was hard. When they received news from there, it was not always positive. If it was not about inflation, it was about a lack of jobs or some other hardship. These reports came so frequently that it was difficult to know why the news about Ebola was different. Besides, only a few people were talking about the outbreak within the African immigrant community. The small size of the Guinean immigrant population made it difficult for information to filter out into the wider African community. This was just how the system worked; news about specific countries mainly circulated within restricted ethnic networks. It only tended to spread to the wider community when things became more serious.

For a long time after the first Ebola-infected persons crossed from Guinea into neighboring countries, the circulation of news about the epidemic continued to be limited. There was no way of predicting that it would become an international crisis. Consequently, many Africans in Dallas continued to travel to Guinea, Liberia, and Sierra Leone with no expectation that life in these countries was about to be disrupted.

The foundations of these movements are rooted in the long tradition of transnational migration between Dallas and West Africa that existed before the start of the epidemic. However, maintaining the transnational connections between the two contexts does not necessarily require migration to and from the region. Improvements in communication have made it easy to maintain social connections with West Africa and enabled immigrants to participate vicariously in the social lives of family members in their origin countries. These two phenomena—migration between Dallas and West Africa and vicarious connections with origin countries—are crucial for understanding how many Africans in Dallas experienced the consequences of the Ebola outbreak in West Africa.

These transnational connections thus provide a basis for developing insights into the various ways in which these immigrants were affected by the spread of the virus in the early stages of the epidemic. Visits to affected countries showed them how societies react when dealing with a deadly epidemic. It required the management of their own fears and the development of measures to avoid the risk of infection. It also warranted the need to prepare for the challenges of life after returning to the United States. In other words, those returning from affected countries needed to grapple with the suspicions of others in Dallas, who were concerned that they had brought the virus with them on their return from West Africa.

But one did not need to travel to the affected countries to experience the early consequences of the epidemic. Staying connected to relatives back home also required the management of anxieties and the development of strategies to respond to the growing threats to their health. And in the worst of circumstances, there was a need to deal with Ebola deaths among loved ones. Responding to this was quite different from responding to deaths under normal circumstances. For example, the former was exacerbated by the impossibility of returning home to perform customary mourning rites. Altogether, the diverse perspectives linked to the implications of transnational connections between Ebola-affected countries and Africans in Dallas are important and critical for demonstrating that their traumatic experiences during the 2014 Ebola epidemic predated the death of Thomas Duncan.

Very rarely do we get to observe the early disruptions caused by epidemics in one world region on the lives of immigrants in another. Yet, the early spread of Ebola from Guinea to its neighboring countries gave us an opportunity to examine the implications of these disruptions for the lives of Africans in Dallas. These disruptions were geographically experienced as a result of African immigrants' social and emotional investments in their origin countries. Thus, it is important to link these experiences across global spaces to develop a comprehensive picture that shows the complex

ways in which epidemics can influence the lives of immigrants. To illumi-
nate these experiences, several questions need to be answered, such as:
What explained the spread of the epidemic from the rural communities
where it started to the urban communities usually visited by Africans in
Dallas? How did perceptions about Ebola affect their decisions to travel to
affected countries? How did those who visited affected countries survive the
early onslaught of the epidemic? And, finally, how did Africans in Dallas
cope with bereavement and loss as the number of Ebola deaths increased?

Reacting to the Spreading Epidemic in West Africa

The first suspicions of Ebola transmission beyond the borders of Guinea
emerged with unconfirmed reports that there was a Sierra Leonean guest
at the Ouamouno family home at the time of Emile's infection. According
to WHO, this person died after returning to Sierra Leone in early January
2014, but their cause of death was undetermined (WHO 2015c). The first
official case of Ebola in the country was confirmed a few months later, after
which subsequent transmissions occurred in a series of super-spreader
events. These events occur when a virus is transmitted from an infected
individual to a disproportionately larger number of people than would
otherwise be expected. A number of studies indicate that super-spreader
events were responsible for most of the infections that occurred during
the epidemic (Stein 2011; Wong et al. 2015).

One of the most significant of these events took place in Sierra Leone.
It involved a traditional healer in the border town of Koidu who was so
renowned that her clients included sick people from Guinea, who traveled
to the country to secure her services. She died of a mysterious illness some-
time in May 2014, and because she was very well known, many people
traveled to Koidu from other parts of Sierra Leone to attend her funeral.
The mourners included thirteen women who were among the first group
of people to die from Ebola in the country (Reuters 2014b). However, the
spread of the disease did not end with them. Another set of Ebola cases was
soon found in Kenema, a town located approximately seventy miles from
Koidu. It consisted of seventy-eight people whose infections were traced
to their interactions with mourners who had attended the funeral in Koidu.
They were admitted to the main government hospital in the town (Gire et
al. 2014; McNeil 2014). By the time most of these chains of transmission

were identified, more than three hundred people were confirmed to have had Ebola infections traced to the traditional healer's death (Fox 2017).

It is possible that similar events were responsible for the early spread of the virus in Liberia. After the first two cases of Ebola in the country were discovered in March 2014, there were strong reasons to suspect that they were linked to the individuals' prior contact with infected persons from Guinea (Davis 2014). In these cases, the individuals are believed to have entered the country from Guinea, through Lofa County in Liberia, which was not far from the source of the epidemic in Meliandou (Ladner et al. 2015). Despite what we know about the first super-spreader events in Sierra Leone, studies of similar events in Liberia are largely unavailable. However, eyewitness accounts of the outbreak in Lofa can give us a glimpse into the social circumstances under which the first set of transmissions are likely to have occurred.

Moses, an immigrant from Liberia who moved to Dallas after the epidemic, was one of the few people in the city present in Lofa when the first Ebola cases were confirmed. Trained as an electrical engineer, he worked as a consultant with a leading UN agency. His main job was to help install solar panels on the new Ebola centers established in the country. On his first assignment, he was part of a team sent by the Liberian government and its UN partners to investigate unconfirmed reports that people infected with Ebola were crossing into Liberia. The reports were coming from the town of Foya, in Liberia's Lofa County, so this is where the team set up work to investigate.

Foya is on the Liberian side of the tri-border region, and it is a market town that lies in close proximity to the Nzérékoré Region in Guinea, where the Ebola epidemic started. One of the first things that stood out to Moses after he arrived was the connectedness of the communities found around the border. According to him, they were so seamlessly linked that "you wouldn't even know that there is a border out there." As a market town, Foya's main economic activity revolved around trade conducted by farmers from nearby communities. Trade was most beneficial to communities on the Liberian side of the border, because they were highly dependent on the goods that were brought to the town from Guinea and Sierra Leone, such as meat, vegetables, and other types of produce. However, a major problem in the area was a lack of reliable healthcare services. As Moses explained, the only source of available healthcare services was a clinic located close to Foya that was constructed to serve employees of a farming project funded by the government of Libya. From Moses's perspective, this clinic was most likely the place that treated the first Ebola-infected persons in Liberia. As the only provider of modern healthcare services in that part of the tri-border region, it usually treated farmers from Guinea and Sierra Leone who came to Foya to sell their produce.

In Foya itself, few people grasped the serious nature of the consequences of Ebola after the first cases were confirmed. According to Moses, their overall level of indifference was astounding, and this paved the way for the subsequent spread of the epidemic to Monrovia. As he explained:

> When I saw how people were behaving in Foya, I knew we had a serious problem. Most people did not think this was something serious. They thought it was a joke. You tell people to do things, to take precautions against the disease, but they respond as if what you are saying is not true. They did not believe anything that was going on. . . . When I went back to Monrovia, I told my friends that the way things are going the disease is going to kill more than a hundred people. They too did not think it was that serious. They were saying, "Oh no, this thing would not kill more than thirty people." However, as I was reading about it and its effects, I thought to myself, "If this thing gets to Monrovia, it would be a complete disaster."

This cynicism about the consequences of Ebola reflected a lack of familiarity with a virus that was largely foreign to the area. It was difficult for people to conceive of the deadly consequences of a disease to which they had never been exposed. In this part of West Africa, communities had hunted the same wild animals, used the same farming methods, and experienced the same patterns of illness over the course of several centuries (WHO 2015c).

It did not take long for the virus to spread beyond the tri-border region to the interiors of Liberia and Sierra Leone. Compared to the Central African countries where Ebola outbreaks had previously occurred, the geography of this region was different. It had lush vegetation around which there were historical pathways of migration that linked these interior communities with coastal settlements in the south. Three of the pathways were still being used for internal migration (Richards 2016). The first followed the northern rivers of Sierra Leone into the interior districts of Guinea. The next two started on either side of the Gola Forest, which is located on the border of Liberia and Sierra Leone, and continued through a forest–savanna zone. On the Liberian side of the forest, one of these routes is connected to major transportation networks leading to Monrovia, while on the Sierra Leonean side, the other route is linked to transportation networks leading to Freetown. It is by way of these routes that the virus spread from the tri-border region to urban centers in Guinea, Liberia, and Sierra Leone during the early phases of the epidemic (Richards 2016).

The reluctance to take precautions against the virus made it easier for the virus to spread along these routes and put communities along their paths at risk (Richards 2016). Compounding these effects was the early indifference of the governments of the affected countries. In Guinea, the government had a strained relationship with the forest communities where the epidemic originated, which made it difficult to break new infection chains as they were being developed (Richards 2016). In Liberia and Sierra Leone, things were slightly different and more directly tied to bad governance. In Liberia, for example, no attempt was made to develop a public information campaign to warn people about the consequences of Ebola during the first few months of the epidemic (Bah and Dosso 2014). In Sierra Leone, the government also made no meaningful effort to combat the virus after early cases were identified in Koidu. After the first cases were confirmed in the capital city several weeks later, a national secretariat was established to lead the campaign against the virus (Garrett 2014).

Notwithstanding the linear patterns of transmission observed during the early stages of the outbreak, the subsequent spread of the virus occurred in spatially random patterns that were difficult to predict. The two Liberian counties most affected by the epidemic, Margibi and Montserrado, were not close to the source of the epidemic, near its northeastern border with Guinea; instead, they were located farther away in Monrovia, in the country's southwest (Ladner et al. 2015). Similarly, in Sierra Leone, the most affected districts were clustered not only close to the tri-border region in the east but also in districts in the northeast (WHO 2016b). Random patterns of diffusion were likewise observed in Guinea, where clusters of affected communities were found in Forecaria, Sigwiri, and Dureka, all of which are located away from the source of the epidemic. By June 2014, the virus had reached most of the major urban centers where many Africans in Dallas usually reside during their visits to the region. However, the toll of the epidemic was much higher in Liberia and Sierra Leone. Indeed, the overall number of deaths due to Ebola at the end of the epidemic was much larger in Liberia and Sierra Leone than it was in Guinea (WHO 2016a).*

Negotiating Safety during the Epidemic at Home

New Ebola cases found in diverse West African regions posed a significant challenge to sustaining the transnational ties that linked immigrants from these countries living in Dallas to their communities of origin. Although these connections can be maintained using the tools of modern communication, there was no substitute for what could be accomplished by being physically present in Africa. Investments could be better monitored, parents could be cared for, and social networks could be cultivated in preparation for eventual resettlement. These demands are better fulfilled when accompanied by a personal touch or physical interaction, or by showing up to confirm your commitment.

However, during the early stages of the epidemic, the risk of traveling to affected countries was significant. It meant that the likelihood of being infected needed to be taken into consideration when determining whether being present at home was *really* that important. Each person had to decide how to react to reports that the virus was spreading outside the border region. Before the epidemic reached major urban centers, their long distance from the border communities where it started created some sense of security. As a result, people continued to travel to Guinea, Liberia, and Sierra Leone during the first few months of the epidemic. There was also a small number of immigrants who were already in the affected countries at the start of the epidemic. Along with the new arrivals, they too needed to consider how to respond to the new risks associated with the spread of the epidemic.

Before turning attention to how immigrants adapted to life under these circumstances, it is important to examine their reasons for traveling to

* Estimates indicate that by the end of 2015, the total number of confirmed cases was 3,804 in Guinea, 10,666 in Liberia, and 14,122 in Sierra Leone. The total number of Ebola deaths was 2,236 in Guinea, 4,806 in Liberia, and 3,955 in Sierra Leone (WHO 2016a).

these high-risk environments during this period. For James, a pastor of a Liberian church near Dallas, it was to conduct a Christian missions trip that was already planned for early 2014. He had a history of making periodic visits to the country. However, it was while visiting Liberia in 2014 that he first heard about the Ebola outbreak. As he recalled what happened during his visit, he was still dismayed by the lack of urgency shown by the government in its initial response: "I was in Liberia. Was it? . . . Yeah, early 2014. We took a missions trip to Liberia. We usually go back once a year. When we were in Monrovia, however, we heard about it, but it was like it was downplayed. In 2014, in March, when we came back to the States, I think then, we started hearing more about Ebola. I think it broke. . . . It really got really bad in the summer of 2014."

Conversely, Tom visited Sierra Leone as part of a personal commitment to make two or more visits to the country each year. He was a highly educated professional working for a school system in Dallas, and he strongly believed in using his resources to advance the plight of the poor. During his first visit in 2014, his main objective was to supervise a project he supports that promotes the education of children with special needs. The first official Ebola diagnosis in the country occurred while he was in Freetown, and two things defined his recollection of how the event specifically unfolded. The first was the uncertainty created by rumors of the spreading virus, even before the first case in the country was confirmed, while the second was his complete ignorance about the deadly virus that formed the basis of these rumors. As he put it: "I was actually there when it started. Toward the end of April, we began to hear rumors that the epidemic had reached the country. In May, we heard that Ebola had reached Lungi. Honestly, I did not know anything about Ebola, so I was one of those people who did not do anything about it. However, by then it was not within the limits of the capital city. It was far away from Freetown."

At this stage, ignorance about Ebola was also highly prevalent among Africans in Dallas who were planning to visit countries affected by the virus. As a result, the perceived threat of the virus was minimal, and many people continued to visit these countries even after the first cases were confirmed. For instance, Tom visited Sierra Leone at least two more times after learning that Ebola cases had occurred in the country. Similarly, there were others in the Liberian immigrant community who made multiple visits to Liberia after learning about the start of the outbreak. Traveling under these circumstances was in some ways counterintuitive, but it also reflected the low assessments of risk that were driven by the lack of information on the virus available at the time.

Others exercised more caution when making their travel decisions and only decided to visit after securing additional information. As Nancy, a nurse in Dallas, acknowledged, she was initially reluctant to travel to Sierra Leone in early 2014 because of what she was hearing about the epidemic. Her original plan was to travel to the country as part of a team that conducted annual visits to provide healthcare services to poor communities in Freetown. Final preparations for the trip had been made at a conference in Europe, where she met with other healthcare workers who were part of her team. Before gathering to make a final decision, they received periodic updates on the spread of the virus, many of which were troubling. Moreover, friends in the country sent Nancy emails that raised serious doubts about whether she should visit that year. The longer they waited to decide, the more she wavered. She described her thoughts at that time as follows: "I was like, 'God, should I really go? Should we call this off?'" The tipping point came after a phone call she received from someone in Sierra Leone. During the call, she learned that although an Ebola case had been found in Lungi, Freetown, the town they were planning to visit, was still Ebola-free. On the basis of this information, the team decided to travel to Sierra Leone as planned, and they left the country before the epidemic got worse.

Not everyone made such decisions. Many others considered the risk of visiting affected countries to be too high to justify a decision to travel. Among them were individuals who had planned celebrations and other big events in West Africa but decided to postpone them until the situation improved. The best example of this was some members of a Krio ethnic organization in Dallas. They had planned to travel to Sierra Leone in December 2014 to host an international homecoming celebration, and plans for the occasion had been initiated two years before the start of the outbreak. These plans included having a meeting with the country's president, organizing a picnic, and conducting a thanksgiving service while in the country. Some members of the organization had even booked their flights earlier in the year, while others booked their flights after the outbreak was confirmed. They did so believing that the virus would be contained before the end of the year. However, in August 2014 it became clear that the epidemic was getting worse, and as a result the trip was postponed.

The people who spent time in the affected countries during the epidemic represent a unique group of individuals with a high tolerance for risk. Living through the chaos of the epidemic was a different matter. It required that several issues be addressed. First, personal fears needed to be acknowledged. Individuals traveling to affected countries had to consider what an Ebola infection meant for their survival as well as their chances of returning to Dallas. In other words, it was important to mitigate the risk of unknowingly returning with the virus, only to begin showing symptoms after its three-week incubation period. Second, it was necessary to develop responses to help these people adapt to the social realities of the epidemic. New habits had to be formed to avoid crowed places, adhere to curfews, and reduce the risk of interacting with possibly infected persons.

As the situation deteriorated, the most immediate concern was to adapt to the new measures taken by the government to combat the spread of the virus. These measures discouraged physical interaction in public places and promoted frequent handwashing with a mixture of water and chlorine. The public was also warned to avoid shaking hands and giving hugs in an effort to break possible chains of infection. As the number of infected persons increased, the local signs of the epidemic also became more visible. Healthcare workers wearing personal protective equipment such as gloves, helmets, and googles while caring for infected individuals were frequently seen on the news, and as Ebola deaths increased, it also became common to see burial workers in protective equipment as they transported corpses to local cemeteries.

Other, more dramatic measures to contain the virus were instituted as the situation deteriorated even further. More communities with affected counties were quarantined, with those with particularly high numbers of new cases being guarded by military forces to ensure that residents stayed within their neighborhoods. This turned out to be very contentious in places where the new measures were unpopular. In Monrovia, for example, residents in the community of West Point were quarantined after multiple Ebola cases were diagnosed in the area. Angry residents who thought this was unfair staged a riot and blamed the spread of the virus within their community on the government's decision to locate an Ebola treatment center in the area. It took troops from the national army to quell the subsequent unrest and enforce a blockade that kept residents of West Point from moving to other communities (Passewe et al. 2014; Quist-Acton 2014).

Apart from these measures, all schools and colleges in the countries that were most affected by the virus were closed to reduce the risk of Ebola transmission among students. Furthermore, in Liberia, markets were either closed or allowed to operate on a limited schedule, while nonessential government workers were sent on mandatory leave (Butty 2014; O'Carroll 2014). Some of these measures were also taken in Sierra Leone. In addition, Sierra Leone's government imposed a national curfew that restricted all public travel to the period between 9 a.m. and 5 p.m. (Nurse and Guest 2015; O'Carroll 2014). Additionally, on multiple occasions more than half of the country's population was quarantined to allow health workers to check houses for infected persons and to bury people suspected to have died from the virus (O'Carroll 2014).

Most Africans visiting from Dallas took these new developments in stride. But this belied the fact that their fears about the fatal consequences of the disease were increasing. These fears were a major motivation for visitors to develop strategies to protect themselves from infection during their time away from the United States. Interestingly, the strategies developed preempted many of the methods later used by Africans in Dallas to address their fear of Ebola during the crisis in the city.

Sam experienced this heightened sense of caution while visiting Liberia, and this was in part fueled by his determination to return to the United States alive. Although he left Liberia during the civil war in the 1990s, he visited in early 2014 to prepare the groundwork for his permanent return in the coming years. The visit was also significant because he used it to travel to neighboring Sierra Leone. He had lived there for a brief time in the 1990s, during which he met a friend who would later become his wife.

Beginning to describe his experiences in both countries, Sam confessed that "it was scary." Nevertheless, he tried to provide some comfort to his hosts, stating that things would be fine if they "just stayed away from close bodily contact with other people." Explaining things further, he described how he became proactive in protecting himself by changing how he used public transportation services. His strategy was simple, but it allowed him to circumvent the system common in Liberia and other African countries that requires that all passengers using a taxicab pay separate fares for the ride. One implication of this approach is that it encourages cabdrivers to maximize their income by getting as many passengers as possible into the cab at one time so that there are no empty seats as they drive between destinations. Therefore, to avoid physical contact with other passengers, Sam employed a strategy he referred to as "doubling up." It reflected the combined influence of his desire to mitigate Ebola infection and his interpretation of the recommendation to avoid physical contact with others. He explained the strategy as follows: "When I got into a taxi, I paid for myself and for the seat next to me. I didn't want anybody leaning on me. If I got the front seat, that was great, because I knew the driver was not going to lean on me, so that's just what I did. Even when I was going to Freetown, I made sure I paid for myself and for the extra seat in a cab that took me all the way from Monrovia to Freetown. I just paid. I didn't want anybody's sweat touching me."

Visiting Sierra Leone allowed Sam to witness much of the confusion that characterized the early phase of the epidemic. He observed the skepticism expressed by people who questioned the existence of a virus they had never heard of. He was particularly struck by their willingness to riot on the basis of this skepticism. For example, some youths threatened to burn down a government hospital in Kenema if Ebola patients admitted there were not released. The youths took this action after hearing from a former nurse who incorrectly informed crowds at a local market that the virus was a gimmick designed to lure patients into hospitals where they would be used for cannibalistic rituals (Fofana 2015). While Sam did not express belief in these claims, his own views about the virus appear to have become less defined by his exposure to these skeptics. As such, he believed that some patients who were diagnosed with Ebola were not really affected by the virus.

More generally, the concern about the need to avoid contact with infected persons was found not only among those visiting the affected countries but also among their hosts. For example, relatives of people visiting from the United States quietly feared that their family members would not be able to return to the States if they became infected. Consequently, they took measures to provide additional layers of protection to further mitigate the risk of infection among their guests.

In the case of Tom, who arrived in Sierra Leone before the start of the epidemic, this parental intervention was done out of concern that he did not appreciate the seriousness of the crisis. He had been reluctant to make major changes in his interactions with others after the first Ebola case was confirmed in Freetown. In fact, the only change he made was to stop shaking hands with others. In his father's opinion, however, that was not enough. As a result, his father took additional steps to protect Tom, for example, by changing his boarding arrangements to minimize his contact with his brothers at home, who frequently spent time out with their friends.

The family compound where Tom stayed had two houses. The first was the main residence—a large house located in the front—and the second was a smaller house in the rear. To restrict Tom's interaction with his brothers, Tom's father devised a strategy that had them living in separate houses in the compound. Tom was asked to remain in the larger house, and a new lock was installed on the front door to deny access to his brothers, while his brothers were asked to move to the smaller house. While Tom did not think the Ebola threat warranted the separate living arrangements, he understood why his dad made the decision. The rationale was simple:

[My dad] did this because [my brothers] were always going out at night and going in and out of the house; he wanted to protect me. I was the golden goose that laid the golden egg, because I send money for them from the US very frequently. So my dad wanted to protect me and do what he could to ensure that I would return safely [laughs]. He himself said that he believed that I was like the pillar of the family and that he was not worried about my younger brothers. This was why he also locked the front door of the house.

Returning to the United States and the Continuing Response to the Epidemic

Back in Dallas, it was slowly becoming obvious that the epidemic was taking a turn for the worse. Those with relatives visiting Africa were becoming increasingly concerned by news reports detailing the gruesome consequences of the epidemic. Dead bodies were being left on the streets, as people refused contact with corpses of people believed to have died of Ebola. Additionally, all private burials were banned to allow trained burial teams to pick up and dispose of all corpses. However, the number of burial workers was not always sufficient to allow for prompt disposal of corpses. Apart from this, things were getting worse economically. The prices of basic necessities were increasing as a result of the artificial scarcity of food. Few food staples were available at local markets because many roads linking farms to urban markets were closed to control the movement of people (Sy and Copley 2014). Another source of concern was the state of decline of healthcare systems in West Africa. It was clear that if relatives visiting the region were infected by the virus, there was only a slim chance that they would receive the treatment they needed to survive.

As these fears increased, those visiting affected countries started to receive calls from friends and family in the United States requesting that they return immediately. In Tom's case, the calls came from friends and members of his church. Yet, it was not easy to respond with the same sense of urgency as that expressed by people calling from Dallas. Returning to Dallas was not just a matter of boarding the next available flight out of Africa. Moreover, perceptions of the threat posed by Ebola differed between individuals visiting Africa and friends who were calling from the States. Therefore, when Tom's friends asked him to return to the United States immediately, he thought they were overreacting. After a friend found his response to be unsatisfactory, he sent Tom $300 to cover the cost of changing the return date on his ticket.

Since transnational movements involve the circulation of migrants between countries, they can sometimes increase the odds that migrants exposed to infections in epidemic contexts will transmit diseases to their communities after they return (Käferstein et al. 1997). Fortunately, none of the Africans in Dallas who traveled to the countries affected during the crisis were infected with the virus. However, returning to Dallas created two new challenges to the resumption of life in the African community. First, those returning had to deal with the lingering suspicion that they may have been infected with the virus but had not yet started showing symptoms. Second, they had to respond to subtle patterns of stigma that challenged the long tradition of bounded solidarity within the African immigrant community.

Alim's experiences are critical to understanding the complications involved in dealing with these challenges. As a member of the Mandingo ethnic group, he was one of many Liberians living in Dallas who also had ancestral roots in Guinea. During his visit to Guinea in early 2014, he decided to make a short trip to neighboring Liberia before returning to the United States. The first Ebola case in Liberia was identified after he arrived in Conakry, Guinea. However, he ignored this development and proceeded with his journey to Liberia. He started his journey by road but had to turn back at the border after the Liberian government banned all movements between the two countries.

Alim returned to Conakry, where he spent some more time before leaving for the United States. Upon his return, he traveled with a young child he had volunteered to bring to her parents in the States. The child looked well enough to travel except for the fact that she was frequently using the bathroom. After they arrived at the airport, they followed the new procedures that required all passengers to wash their hands with a mixture of water and chlorine before boarding. New York was Alim's final transit point before returning to Dallas, and it was also where the girl was supposed to be picked up by her parents. However, shortly after arriving Alim started to feel sick. His first thought was that something must have gone wrong in Guinea to make him sick, but he could not identify what it was. His attention then turned to his traveling companion, and for the first time during their time together, he became concerned that the young child may have infected him with Ebola. Describing these events, Alim observed the following:

> I was sick. I was feeling sick because . . . you know, you feel like you're not feeling well. I was very scared because I came with a little girl, and she had an upset stomach. Her grandparents had asked me to travel with her and bring her to her parents. But they too were concerned that the little girl had an upset stomach. We gave her Flagyl to stop her diarrhea, but I mean, I was kind of scared being around her. When I got to New York, I called her dad and he was there to pick up his daughter. Looking back, [what I was feeling] had nothing to do with Ebola, but my mind kept telling me that it did, although the little girl just had diarrhea.

Alim's experience was not unique. He explained that he also had a friend who became ill after returning to the United States from Liberia.

This friend lived with him for a few days after arriving in Dallas but told no one he was ill. When he called from a hospital to inform Alim that he was there to see a doctor, Alim was surprised, but he was not too concerned because his friend assured him that he did not have Ebola. Word soon got out to others in the community that there was a sick man from Liberia staying at Alim's house. Subsequently, Alim started to receive calls from people expressing their disapproval. As he recalled, "People started telling me, 'Man, you better be careful receiving people from Africa. A number of people are coming here sick, and this [Ebola] thing is spreading very fast.'" At this point, there had been no confirmed cases of Ebola among people arriving in Dallas from West Africa. Nevertheless, there was already a growing belief that those returning from affected countries should be avoided because they could potentially infect others with the virus.

Alim allowed his friend to continue to stay at his house mainly because of his own experiences after returning to the United States. After arriving in New York, he spent two days with friends before finally returning to Dallas. He did not forget that his friends remained hospitable to him even when they knew that he was sick. Later, they informed him that although they were concerned that he was possibly infected with Ebola, they allowed him to stay with them because he was someone they could trust.

The implications of this experience were clear. These were times when people thought they needed to be careful about hosting guests who were returning from countries affected by the virus. New fears about the consequences of infection meant that community norms on giving mutual assistance needed to be reassessed. The difficulties involved in differentiating who was infected by the virus from who was not posed significant strains on the community's bonds of solidarity. While Alim's experiences suggested that these bonds were not easy to break, they reflected the start of new social changes that were stemming from the increased awareness of Ebola among Africans in the city.

Embracing the Realities of Ebola in Dallas

News about the epidemic started to spread within the African community at a time when few people in Dallas had heard about the Ebola virus. These included many immigrants from the affected countries who had never lived through an Ebola epidemic. Firsthand reports of travelers' experiences in these countries helped increase awareness of the disruptions caused by the virus. However, it took time for networks of information transmission within the community to become sufficiently saturated with these reports and for the consequences of the epidemic to be taken more seriously.

Reactions to the new developments were diverse. Except for immigrants from countries where prior Ebola outbreaks had occurred, few people grasped the magnitude of the public health crisis that was unfolding in West Africa. Among the few people who knew something about the virus was someone who recalled hearing about it several years before while watching an episode of *The Bernie Mac Show*. In that episode, Bernie Mac was concerned that his children were sick because they were coughing in their bedroom. And expressing his surprise, he turned to his wife and yelled, "They've got Ebola!" to prevent his wife from entering the room.

With increasing US media coverage of the epidemic, more people were curious to learn about the virus. Accordingly, when Aisha, an immigrant from Sierra Leone, heard about it for the first time, she decided to conduct her own investigations to understand why so many people were concerned. The first time she heard about the virus was on the evening news, and she described her reaction as follows:

> After I heard them talking about Ebola on the news, I said to myself, "What's that?" They then started saying that this was a deadly disease. But I still had no idea what this was. So I called my sister in Sierra Leone and asked her, "What is Ebola?" She said to me, "I'm telling you . . . this is a deadly thing. I have stopped visiting people and going to places where I really don't need to be. To be safe, we now have to protect our clothes, wash them with bleach and hang them up, before we can wear them." . . . [It was] after this that I started reading news stories about the doctor who died in Sierra Leone.

The doctor Aisha was referring to was Sheik Umar Khan. He was the leading specialist in viral hemorrhagic fever in Sierra Leone, and his death increased international media attention on the crisis. Dr. Khan's role in the response to the epidemic is considered by many to be heroic. He provided care to some of the first victims of the virus and inadvertently became infected during the process. He later became the first doctor in the country to die from Ebola. Because his death occurred around the same time that

Dr. Brantly became infected with Ebola, news coverage of both events helped to reinforce the seriousness of the crisis to many Africans in Dallas. However, at this point there was very little they could do. One Sierra Leonean organization in the city tried to explore the possibility of bringing Dr. Khan to the United States for treatment, but a day after these plans were initiated, he died at an Ebola treatment center in Sierra Leone.

As more people learned about Ebola and its consequences, new questions began to emerge about the origins of the virus. How did it get to a part of Africa where such an epidemic had never been seen before? Was the virus really the cause of so many deaths in such a short period of time? Skeptical questions about the origins of disease are not new. In fact, there is a long history of expressions of skepticism about the causes of disease during times of health crises. After the start of the AIDS epidemic, for example, there was a growing number of skeptics dedicated to spreading conspiracy theories about the origins of the virus (Kalichman 2009). Research on the Zika virus similarly indicates that in some cases conspiracy theories are more popular than accurate information disseminated by the media (Sharma et al. 2017). Another characteristic of these theories is that they are usually found not just among the uneducated but among trained scientists and medical personnel as well (Goertzel 2010; Maridor, Bangerter, and Emery 2017).

A popular strand of skepticism about the origins of the Ebola epidemic was claiming that the virus had man-made origins that could be traced to the West. Among the leading proponents of this view was Cyril Broderick, a Liberian professor who taught at Delaware State University. He published an article in the *Daily Observer* in Liberia that made several claims about the origins of the Ebola crisis (Broderick 2014). He maintained that the virus was a genetically modified organism created in the United States and suggested that it was being tested in Guinea and Sierra Leone shortly before the start of the epidemic. Broderick was thus concerned that the timing of the Ebola outbreak apparently coincided with reports of the arrival of US scientists in the affected countries to conduct research. His views received widespread coverage in Liberia. While many of his claims were contested by commentators (e.g., Kincaid 2014; Lowe 2014), they still found a sympathetic audience in Liberia and among African immigrants in the diaspora (McCoy 2014).

Some Africans in Dallas thus invoked Broderick's claims as they questioned the roots of the epidemic occurring in their origin countries. The skeptical views were found in claims such as "America created it" and in less definitive assertions such as "We heard that someone was doing research in West Africa around this time. So we don't know whether this virus was made by Western scientists." Also related to these suspicions was the belief that if Ebola was native to West Africa, prior evidence of its existence would have been found in the region's forests. Expressing this line of thought, one immigrant asked rhetorically: "Where was Ebola since it was found in the DRC? Was it in monkeys all these years and gradually killing them?" From his perspective, it was difficult to believe that the virus could have existed among animals in the region because, as he subsequently affirmed, people would have seen many dead animals in the jungles of West Africa. Because evidence for this was lacking, he argued that the only alternative explanation for the start of the outbreak was that it had man-made origins.

Partly fueling these suspicions was the perceived inconsistency between the traditional narrative on the causes of Ebola, which emphasized its zoonotic origins, and cultural traditions found in many parts of rural Africa. Some of the skeptics maintained that the relationship between the typical causes of an Ebola infection and the consumption of bush meat was implausible. Dismissing this relationship as fictional, one skeptic observed the following: "We've been eating bush meat for a very long time, but we have never had an epidemic. Ebola did not kill us. How can this outbreak start all of a sudden when it never existed in the country before?"

Despite these doubts, there was a consensus that something needed to be done. Driven by the spate of deaths among doctors and other healthcare professionals, several African immigrant organizations started to explore options for what they could do. There was a wide range of issues that needed to be addressed, and it was too early to identify areas of priority. However, it was clear that public health systems in countries affected by the virus were so deplorable that they were incapable of handling such a crisis. After all, this was why many immigrant organizations in Dallas provided support to the healthcare sector in various West African countries—even before the start of the epidemic. There were also concerns about the perceived culture of complacency. Reflecting Moses's concerns about the lack of urgency in containing the virus in Foya, the general opinion was that getting people to change their habits would be difficult. As one immigrant surmised: "I was worried because some of [our people] even have problems with simple hygiene, so I was thinking, 'Hey, this thing is going to spread all over.'"

As they learned more about prior Ebola epidemics in other parts of Africa, some immigrant leaders from affected countries became increasingly outraged that their governments were not moving fast enough to tackle the crisis. Why did Liberia and Sierra Leone wait so long to close their borders with Guinea? This, many believed, represented a failure to learn from the experiences of Uganda and the DRC. In these two countries, authorities typically take prompt action to contain Ebola outbreaks to prevent the spread of the virus to larger urban areas. Community leaders with highly placed contacts in Liberia and Sierra Leone thus believed that they needed to spur their governments into action by lobbying them to do more.

Abu, an activist from Sierra Leone with ties to the Liberian immigrant community, was involved in these efforts, which he argued were more organized among Liberians. He was part of a group of West African professionals who worked with leaders in the Liberian community to plan lobbying activities. He described how conference calls were used to develop strategies for determining how their collective influence could be used to encourage more rapid governmental action in the affected countries. During one such call, some of the leaders used their contacts in Liberia to facilitate a phone conversation between the group and a senior Liberian government official. Of the discussions, Abu recalled the following:

> [We] were able to talk to the then . . . I think she was the Minister of Education or Health in Liberia. Incidentally, she did much of [her] schooling in Sierra Leone, and before her appointment to the government she was a popular singer in both countries. I engaged her in a conversation, and my first question to her was "Why did you guys not first reach out to the people with experience addressing these issues in Uganda and the DRC to learn from them rather than wait for the international community to bring aid?" And her response was, "Well, [Abu], you know the situation in Africa. We don't really move as fast as we should."

While the official's candor was appreciated, it also confirmed their worst fears. These fears were discussed in terms of the lost opportunities for curbing the virus. But latent in them was the critical question of what governmental inaction could imply for the survival of their families. By then, the virus was rapidly spreading to the urban centers that many immigrants called home. And in the absence of a stronger response to control the spread of the virus to these cities, the consequences for their relatives at home seemed bleak. As much as being in Dallas provided a semblance of protection from the threat of the epidemic, the fear that the virus was about to strike close to home was real, and it created significant anxiety about what would happen next.

Bereavement and Loss Due to Ebola

Compared to the few people with friends who visited West Africa during the first phases of the epidemic, there was a larger number of immigrants from affected countries with relatives who still lived in the region. As reports of the devastation caused by the virus increased, attention soon turned to the fate of those who were left behind. Unconfirmed rumors about the communities to which the epidemic was spreading only served to heighten these concerns. However, there was very little these immigrants could do other than call family members at home to reiterate the message of caution and to remind them to stay indoors as much as possible. Concerns regarding the ensuing economic hardships were easier to handle. Money could be sent back home through wire transfers as a way to provide the resources needed to cope with the consequences of inflation. But it did not take long for the limits of these efforts to become clear. The first reports began to arrive confirming the deaths of relatives due to Ebola, which shattered all hope that the fatal consequences of the epidemic could be avoided. Moreover, these reports put the bereaved in the difficult predicament of not immediately knowing how to respond.

It is not often that the ways in which immigrants respond to such tragedies are documented in the literature. Moreover, there is very limited research examining how their responses to traumatic events unfold during global epidemics. However, to begin the analysis of these responses among Africans in Dallas, it is important to situate the significance of their bereavement within the context of larger cultural processes.

Deaths, births, and other life transitions have powerful meanings in the cultural norms of African societies (Bonsu and Belk 2003; Peddle et al.

1999). However, perceptions of death are important because of its function in the order of life and its significance for linking the present with the past. Rituals performed during the mourning of a loved one are not just ways to come to terms with grief but pathways through which mourners can connect with ancestral traditions. Nonetheless, the specific rituals used in mourning processes vary. In most cases, they require family members to perform specific roles tied to their relationship with the deceased, their stature within the family, and the resources they can provide. Mourning rituals are also sometimes conducted with larger goals in mind. For instance, among some groups in West Africa, funerals are celebrated with the objective of enabling the deceased to reach the elevated status of an ancestor (Fairhead 2014). Others further conduct elaborate forty-day feasts, during which the life of the deceased is celebrated and larger ancestral connections are invoked.

For Africans living abroad, periods of bereavement provide a unique opportunity to reconnect with cultural traditions and to reaffirm their sense of identity (Zirh 2012). However, most of these traditions need to be observed as part of a larger community of mourners, and this typically requires a physical presence at home. This implies that for many Africans, the performance of cultural rituals during periods of bereavement cannot be completed fully while living abroad. In fact, the ceremonies and rituals performed during the mourning process are so important that even immigrants who do not visit home regularly make an effort to return after the death of relatives. If the deceased is a close family member, returning becomes even more important. This is driven by the perception that in such cases the bereaved especially owes a duty to pay last respects to the deceased and to provide him or her with a fitting funeral (Baffoe and Asimeng-Boahene 2013).

Ebola deaths in Africa made it impossible to meet these obligations and as a result created a notable void in the immigrant experience of bereavement. The risk of being infected was too high to justify a decision to return home, leaving many of the bereaved disconnected from their cultural processes of closure. This predicament is somewhat similar to that found in studies on the transnational bereavement processes of undocumented immigrants (Bravo 2017). Like bereaved Africans in Dallas, undocumented immigrants carry a psychological burden of mourning when they are grieving that is accentuated by the fear of being unable to return if they leave to attend funerals in their home countries. Both cases demand that the desire to pay respects to the deceased be balanced by the need for self-preservation, and for many immigrants the inability to reconcile these demands can make them susceptible to depression (Bravo 2017).

The central institutions that led responses to the challenges of transnational bereavement during the Ebola crisis were immigrant churches. Bishop Roberts was one of the people involved in these responses, and he witnessed the personal toll of bereavement among African immigrants after returning to Dallas from Liberia. Much of this occurred while providing counseling services to church members and others in the Liberian immigrant community. The task of providing these services became even more important as the number of bereaved Liberians increased. The emotional toll of counseling the bereaved was more telling when it involved the grieving members of his church. Church services on Sunday increasingly became more about mourning than celebrating. But the rest of the week was no different. Most people in the Liberian community knew how to reach the bishop by phone, and as a result he continued counseling the bereaved outside regular church service hours.

Reflecting on the challenges he experienced during this period, Bishop Roberts solemnly observed that "as a pastor of Liberian immigrants in this community, I had to deal with a lot. . . . People were coming to me after church in tears because they had just heard that five members of their family had died. I mean, every Sunday. . . . Every day, my phone was ringing. People were calling me saying, 'Pastor, my whole family just got wiped out.' So I usually come here [to his church] and pray for them. After that, I established a more organized process of grief counseling." At one point, the number of bereaved Liberians increased to such an extent that the bishop became stretched beyond his capacity to provide individual counseling. Consequently, he decided to start offering group counseling instead. This shift was important because it allowed him to give more attention to what was happening in Liberia. Upon receiving news that people he knew in Liberia had lost loved ones to Ebola, he made an effort to call from Dallas to provide counseling to them over the phone.

Estimates of how many Africans in Dallas lost loved ones to Ebola during this period are not available. However, as expected, the most frequent reports of these experiences came from Liberians and Sierra Leoneans. Many people from these groups also appeared to know someone in their community who lost family members to Ebola. Indeed, there were enough personal accounts of experiences with bereavement to provide us with a window into the emotional struggles associated with mourning Ebola-related deaths in Africa while living so far away from home.

While speaking about the death of his cousin to Ebola, Alim described the experience as "the worst part of the crisis." It signaled the end of their dreams of a reunion that had led them to begin preparations for Alim's cousin's immigration to the United States. By the early part of 2014, these preparations had become more advanced, and Alim had become financially and emotionally invested. He had sent all the documents his cousin needed to apply for the visa at the American Embassy in Monrovia, and things were looking great. The best sign of this came when the embassy scheduled a date for his cousin to be interviewed. However, a few days before the interview, his cousin became infected with Ebola and died shortly thereafter.

Another person with a compelling experience was Eku, who lost her cousin to Ebola during the epidemic in Sierra Leone. Eku's cousin was one of the country's leading specialist physicians, and, like Dr. Khan, he was infected with the virus while caring for a patient. After starting to show symptoms of Ebola, efforts were made to get him an experimental treatment that would have increased his chances of survival. Unfortunately, however, he died before the treatment arrived. This news devastated Eku, and she was thus emotional as she described why this loss was very personal—she grew up in the same household as her cousin and was so close to him that she considered him a brother.

Still, few accounts were as compelling as Ken's. As a pastor of a church with Liberian and Sierra Leonean members, he provided extensive counseling to congregants who lost family members to Ebola in countries affected by the virus. However, things took a turn for the worse when Ken himself went through one of the most extensive cases of Ebola-related bereavement among Africans in Dallas. In the span of one week, Ken lost two cousins as well as an aunt and her entire family in Liberia. No one had suspected that his aunt was infected with Ebola after she started showing symptoms of an illness. Consequently, she continued living in the same house with relatives who took care of her. A sequence of transmissions then occurred over the course of a few days that resulted in very tragic consequences. As he recalled these events, the teary-eyed pastor explained what had happened: "They were living together, and there was no proper hygiene and education. My aunt's daughter and son contracted it by caring . . . for their mother. My aunt's son, who was my cousin, then spread it to his wife. My cousin, who was my aunt's daughter, who got it from my aunt, then transmitted it to one of her twins. She had twins and she transmitted it to one of the kids . . . and within one week or let me say the space of ten days I lost those five members of my family in Liberia."

Such accounts of personal loss were unquestionably grueling, yet not all experiences of bereavement during this period were directly tied to an Ebola infection. In one case in particular, bereavement was due to the unintended consequences of the new measures adopted in Sierra Leone to combat the spread of the epidemic. Accordingly, the policy of exclusive government control of burials made it all but impossible to provide customary funerals for those who died from other causes. Ola, an immigrant from the country, was thus disappointed because he believed the policy possibly explained why his brother was buried as a pauper. Although his brother's death was due to injuries sustained in an accident, Ola's family was not allowed to perform the customary funeral rites, even after providing evidence to the authorities confirming that his brother's death was due to an injury. As was the case for persons who died from Ebola, his brother was interred by members of the government's burial team. This meant that the corpse was not buried in the plot owned by the family at the cemetery but in one of the inconspicuous spots where victims of the virus were buried.

This incongruence between customary burial norms and the burial practices used during the epidemic was a problem for many in the African community in Dallas. While funerals are supposed to be elaborate events that celebrate the lives of the deceased, official burial teams distinctively strayed from these norms. They transported multiple corpses at a time in the same vehicle, which meant that the deceased did not receive the individual attention their relatives expected them to receive. After burial plots in local cemeteries were exhausted, there was another departure from the norm: the use of cremation to dispose of corpses. This practice is foreign to societies that have long-held traditions about the continuation of life after death (Manguvo and Mafuvadze 2015).

Resistance to nontraditional burial practices was one of the major factors responsible for the early, rapid spread of the virus during the epidemic. In fact, Moses, who worked in Lofa after the first Ebola cases were confirmed, maintained that in some Liberian communities, disapproval of the practice of cremation explained why people kept corpses in their homes rather than hand them over to burial teams. When health officials learned about this, they started to search for corpses from house to house in the most affected areas.

Among many Africans in Dallas, the dual effects of their absence from home and their inability to provide customary burial rights for their loved ones are therefore important for understanding why the grieving process was particularly difficult. It placed them in a difficult position and left them without a solution. It accentuated their feelings of powerlessness and undercut their vicarious social connections. Confronting the process of bereavement during the epidemic thus reinforced the fact that these were not normal times. However, as they would soon discover, their social realities were about to be transformed further. The first Ebola case in America was about to be confirmed, and immigrants would soon learn how to navigate these new experiences within a context of fear, misinformation, and stigma.

Making Sense of the Emerging Crisis Faced by Africans in Dallas

The early stage of the Ebola epidemic is important for examining the diverse experiences of Africans in Dallas during the period preceding the arrival and death of Thomas Duncan. Many experienced the consequences of the crisis before it reached the United States, and their exposure to these consequences was determined by two factors. The first was their countries of origin, and the second was their physical location at the time of the crisis. In terms of the former, these early experiences were almost exclusive to immigrants from affected countries. However, there were notable differences in the ways these consequences were experienced depending on whether individuals were physically present in the affected countries.

Those who visited these countries had firsthand experience living at the center of what would later become the site of a global epidemic. This experience was defined by constant reminders of the threat to their survival, observations of the difficulties involved in curbing an epidemic in resource-poor contexts, and proactive attempts to maximize their survival using different strategies. But those who remained in Dallas were no less affected by the epidemic. Whether it was their concern for friends visiting the region, their apprehensions about governmental inaction, or their experiences with bereavement, they also faced indisputable challenges as they came to terms with the early consequences of the epidemic. Many of these consequences were experienced by their peers who visited West Africa. As such, for immigrants with transnational connections to the affected countries, the question of whether they visited home during the epidemic was not as important in identifying who was affected by the crisis as was understanding how these effects were experienced.

Within the larger African community in Dallas, the early stage of the epidemic was characterized by specific shifts in a number of related social processes. Being embedded in transnational networks connecting Dallas with the Ebola hot spots in Africa created a new basis for considering the risk when deciding whether or not to travel. The desire for self-preservation in the face of fears about Ebola required an honest evaluation of whether their physical presence abroad was truly warranted. While the outcomes of these evaluations differed, the general tendency was to consider these risks of infection too high to warrant travel.

Another shift that occurred was the change in social processes of interaction associated with a return to Dallas after visits to affected countries. Concerns about the health status of returning immigrants necessitated a reassessment of norms regarding the delivery of mutual assistance. One consequence of this was the emergence of subtle signs of stigma among individuals who grappled with their own fears about interacting with people who were possibly infected with the virus. Significantly, however, the new contexts of social interaction did not lead to a breakdown of the traditional bonds of solidarity. It was still possible to provide support to close friends returning to Dallas, even at the expense of putting one's life at risk.

A third change that occurred within the African community was related to the emergence of new obstacles to the practice of customary grieving norms. No longer did the death of loved ones at home provide immigrants with an opportunity to reconnect with cultural traditions. Fears of the likelihood of an Ebola infection similarly outweighed the incentive to travel to meet these obligations. Nothing could have been done to adequately fill the void created by these circumstances. While community resources in the form of immigrant churches played an active role in supporting the bereaved, this was no substitute for the customary rites usually associated with bereavement. For the very first time, therefore, many Africans in Dallas were constrained into a transnational mourning process that left them disconnected from the cultural norms central to their identities.

The emotional burden of the epidemic was still being experienced by immigrants from affected countries when the first case of Ebola was diagnosed in Dallas. This diagnosis ushered them into the next phase of their traumatic experience, which left them vulnerable to the double burden of the crisis. During this phase, national origins became less important for defining African immigrants' experiences, while their personal experiences with stigma became even more extensive.

5 The Tragedy in Dallas

Louise Troh started planning for Duncan's 2014 visit in the fall of 2013. This time the outcome was expected to be different—not like before, when his plans to travel to the United States had been unsuccessful. One of these previous occasions occurred in the late 1990s, after the denial of his application to the US Refugee Resettlement Program. After that, he remained in Ivory Coast while Troh left for the United States with Karsiah, their young son. With the end of Liberia's conflict, Duncan returned home to Liberia, remaining hopeful that he would one day see Karsiah. However, the long period of separation from Troh took its toll, and the relationship between the two ended, and she moved on with her new life in Dallas. Shortly before Karsiah completed high school, however, the relationship between Troh and Duncan was rekindled. As a result, Karsiah's upcoming graduation was the perfect opportunity to resume their plans for a reunion (Troh 2015). To accomplish this goal, Troh took out a loan in the summer of 2014 and used it to purchase Duncan's plane ticket. After that, she waited for his arrival.

In Paynesville, a small town near Monrovia, and with his plane ticket purchased, Duncan accelerated preparations for his visit. However, when he heard that his neighbor was sick, he took time off to offer his assistance. Part of this was because she was more than just a neighbor. She was a relative of his landlord and was also pregnant (Dixon 2014; Sach 2014). No one expected that she was infected with Ebola, even though there was a full-blown epidemic in Monrovia. Thus, her family decided to take her to a clinic to get her treated for what they thought was malaria. Duncan helped her dad and brother carry her to a cab. At the clinic, she was given intravenous fluids, but the fluids did not help (Dixon 2014). Healthcare workers therefore recommended that she be transferred to a larger facility in the city; however, given the upsurge in Ebola patients in Monrovia, neither of the two hospitals they visited were able to admit her. Several hours later, the men brought her back home, and, together, they carried her from the cab to her house and placed her on the floor.

Each stage of the journey involved some kind of interaction between the patient and her helpers, and it was this that set off a chain of contagion that started in Paynesville and continued all the way to Dallas. On their way to the cab, Duncan reportedly held on to her legs while others supported her back (Dixon 2014; Sach 2014). Other reports claim that she vomited on Duncan while he was trying to help (Dixon 2014; Sach 2014). When the woman died later that evening, her body was prepared for burial by people who had no idea that it was plagued with Ebola. Four days later, Duncan departed for the United States, but it was still early in the virus' twenty-one-day incubation period, so he had no visible symptoms. The timing of the departure was important; it meant that he was able to successfully pass screening tests used to identify Ebola-infected persons at the airport in Monrovia. After that, he boarded his flight and headed for the United States.

On September 20, 2014, after arriving in Dallas, the planned reunion between Troh and Duncan finally occurred. It was the ultimate marker of their rekindled relationship and an opportunity for Duncan to reunite with other Liberian immigrants. At Troh's residence in Vickery Meadow, well-wishers and friends stopped by to welcome him to the city. Nothing seemed amiss except that he came down with a fever a few days later. As his health deteriorated, Troh took him to the emergency room at the Texas Health Presbyterian (THP) hospital, which is located near Vickery Meadow. Responding to his reported symptoms of fever and acute abdominal pains, doctors conducted a CT scan and blood tests in an attempt to diagnose his ailment. Based on the results, they concluded that he had a sinus infection and sent him home with antibiotics (Landers 2014; Troh 2015).

It is still unclear whether he told the hospital staff that he had just arrived from West Africa. Some reports claim that he merely told them he was from Africa and that he failed to mention that he helped someone with Ebola a few days earlier (Selk 2014), while others indicate that he did, in fact, mention that he had arrived from Liberia (Troh 2015). Despite these contradictions, one thing is certain: the initial diagnosis did not consider the fact that he had lived in an epidemic environment just before arriving in the United States. Two days later, he returned to the THP hospital in an ambulance looking even sicker than before. This time, the hospital staff treated him with the presumption that he had been infected with Ebola, and as a result, he was admitted and isolated while additional tests were conducted (Landers 2014). It took another couple days for his test results to arrive. They were positive for Ebola, making him the first person to be diagnosed with the disease on US soil.

Duncan's diagnosis had several additional implications. First, it triggered a chain of events that culminated in what was perhaps the largest public health crisis in the United States in the twenty-first century. About a couple weeks after Duncan's diagnosis, two nurses who cared for him at the hospital—Amber Vinson and Nina Pham—were also diagnosed with the virus. Confirmation of this new chain of transmission significantly increased concern that other cases were about to follow. Fortunately, this did not happen. Nevertheless, among the three infected individuals, there were notable differences in the outcomes of their diagnoses, namely, Duncan died several days after his infection was confirmed, and the two nurses recovered. Within the city, fears about the spread of the virus continued to increase and were particularly intense around the three neighborhoods where the three infected persons lived. But nowhere were these fears so heightened than in Vickery Meadow; among other things, it was the disadvantaged community that had long been a major source of concern.

Another implication of Duncan's ordeal was that it cemented the global connection between the epidemic in West Africa and the local outbreak in the city. It demonstrated how difficult it was to contain the spread of an incurable disease from the region to one of the world's most advanced countries. All it took was for one infected person to slip through the screening tests conducted at the airport in Monrovia to create a major public health emergency. As a result, the boundaries of the threat posed by the virus were expanded in ways that made it more immediate to Americans. This made them feel vulnerable, and in view of the systemic failures that made this threat possible, the link between the two Ebola-related events fueled concerns of a looming catastrophe.

Also important was the way the diagnosis influenced how the threat was conceived. It increased focus on the perceived source of the threat, that is, Africans living in close proximity to Americans. This was quite different than the focus that was placed on African immigrants during the HIV/ AIDS epidemic. In the case of the Ebola outbreak, the perceived threat was shaped by several realities. Unlike HIV/AIDS, it could not be avoided by simply making personal choices such as having sex with condoms. More-over, although perceptions of race shaped the focus on African immigrants during both epidemics, their influence on the Ebola outbreak was differ-ent. It was the first time that a definitive link was made between the threat of a foreign killer virus and someone with an African face.

Beyond these issues, the diagnosis was important for generating new re-sponses among Africans in the city. While they had a tradition of respond-ing to various types of crises, that triggered by the new Ebola outbreak was critical. It required them to balance the need to express solidarity with co-ethnics with the need for caution regarding the risks of the virus. It increased the national visibility of Africans in the city, as they received unprecedented exposure in the media. In the process, their leaders were courted by the press in ways that required them to develop new strategies for dealing with all the attention.

More importantly, the Ebola outbreak marked a significant shift in the social experience of the epidemic for all Dallas residents. It was the *proxi-mate* physical event linked to the epidemic. However, for many West Afri-cans it marked the second phase of their experience with the epidemic. This does not imply that they experienced the previous stage, marked by the *distal* physical event, and this new phase sequentially. Continuing trans-national connections between Dallas and West Africa meant that many of them experienced both phases concurrently.

Understanding the social experiences associated with the outbreak re-quires an examination of the factors that determine how Africans and other city residents responded. In some cases, these responses were simi-lar. Both groups, for example, shared concerns about the need to stop the local spread of the virus. In other cases, their responses were different, as in their perceptions of who bore the most responsibility for the outbreak in the city. These perspectives are fundamental for developing a portrait of how immigrant communities reacted to the threat of an epidemic. What were the fears triggered by the start of the outbreak? How did community leaders react to news linking the outbreak to a co-ethnic? To what extent did immigrants use their own experiences to interpret those of Duncan?

In order to develop this portrait, it is also necessary to examine how two other factors influenced how these responses unfolded. The first is racial and ethnic minority status. In part, the significance of race/ethnicity reflects the fact that African immigrants' own racial experiences provided a critical lens through which the crisis was understood. This does not discount the objective question of whether Duncan's ordeal was influenced by systematic patterns of racial discrimination. Rather, it reflects that among these immigrants racial and ethnic frameworks were important for making sense of the contrasting experiences of Duncan and those of the other Ebola-infected Americans. The second factor was low-income status. It recognizes the fact that Duncan was a poor immigrant and that he was hosted by his fiancée, who also had a low socioeconomic position. It is important to understand whether and how both of these factors may have influenced their experiences in the Dallas healthcare system.

Evaluating the Response to the Crisis

More generally, the evaluation of the reaction to the outbreak must begin against the backdrop of discourses on the social response to epidemics. As could be recalled, one of the first responses to these events was the expression of fear (Alcabes 2009; Eichelberger 2007). It has already been noted that the fear of Ebola was highly prevalent among Africans visiting Ebola-affected African countries as well as some in Dallas during the distal physical event. With the outbreak in Dallas, the need to examine the role of this response is once again important. However, as concerns about one's own mortality increase, the search for explanations begins. As such, as fear increases, another response becomes important, that is, the desire to seek attribution or, in other words, to identify the cause of what is happening. In this case, it involved coming to terms with how to locate Duncan within a narrative of blame.

Related to this narrative are new opportunities for evaluating the importance of structural barriers that limit access to health. Once again, race and ethnicity are important bases for assessing the cause of the outbreak, especially given the well-established links between race and access to healthcare. African immigrants' subjective perceptions on these issues are important for evaluating their influence on the crisis, and this is for several reasons. Among them is the fact that for some, these perceptions are rooted in their experiences of discrimination in the healthcare system. Their familiarity with discrimination thus became a basis for understanding Duncan's experiences at the THP hospital and helped to underscore their belief in an inherent bias against Black Africans in the healthcare system.

The fact that these perspectives are subjective does not make them less important. Previous studies indicate that patients from racial and ethnic minority groups know when they are being stereotyped and are able to recognize prejudice and discrimination demonstrated by healthcare personnel (Bird and Bogart 2001). Accordingly, minority patients recognize when they are being treated discourteously or judged unfairly and can link such behaviors to attributes such as their race and class (Bird and Bogart 2001; Johnson et al. 2004). To be sure, these views are limited in their ability to help us assess the objective impact of discrimination on healthcare decisions; however, they are useful in examining how racial minorities understand what they experience during the process of obtaining healthcare from institutional providers (Kressin et al. 2008; Shavers et al. 2012).

Nevertheless, the evidence on the disadvantage associated with race and ethnicity can stand on its own without resorting to the use of subjective perceptions. Compared to Whites, Blacks are less likely to receive major diagnostic or therapeutic procedures, intensive hospital care, and aggressive treatment for ailments including prostate cancer, coronary heart disease, and stroke (Feagin and Bennefield 2014; Harris et al. 1997; Klabunde et al. 1998; Mayberry et al. 2000). Patients from minority populations are also less likely to be treated by specialists or receive simple preventive procedures such as flu vaccines compared to Whites (Blustein and Weiss 1998; Gornick et al. 1996). What this means is that even with the lack of objective evidence on racial inequalities in access to healthcare, it is impossible to ignore the possibility that these factors may, in part, explain why Duncan's experiences were different from those of other Americans.

But the story on inequalities in access to healthcare is not just one about race and ethnicity. Health insurance also matters because it helps reduce individuals' out-of-pocket payments and provides a signal of one's ability to cover the costs of treatment. However, immigrants, racial and ethnic minorities, and other socioeconomically disadvantaged groups have some of the lowest levels of access to health insurance in the country (Derose et al. 2007). Additionally, for foreign visitors such as Duncan, health insurance is usually available through private sources; however, these services are usually expensive.

When such visitors or immigrants from low-income groups become sick, their options for getting healthcare are limited to two options. The first is the use of emergency healthcare services because US law requires hospitals to provide emergency care to all patients regardless of their ability to pay,* and the second is to use the services of federally qualified health centers (FQHCs). These are centers that provide comprehensive health services to low-income and underserved populations, and are reimbursed for services they provide through Medicare or Medicaid.

Given Duncan's lack of health insurance, his healthcare provider options were limited. Close to where he lived in Vickery Meadow, they included the emergency services of the THP hospital, which is a private hospital, and a nearby FQHC. The latter also served most of the neighborhood's large refugee population, and as such it was more familiar with tropical infectious diseases. Of these two choices, however, Duncan chose to go with the former, perhaps because it was closer to Troh's apartment than the alternative provider.

Confusion, Fear, and Duncan's Diagnosis

From his office near Vickery Meadow, Dustin could see the strange buzz of activity near the apartment complex where Troh lived. Dustin was a longtime employee of a refugee resettlement agency and had personally helped resettle refugees in the neighborhood. Gazing out the window of his office, the scene he saw was chaotic. At least four helicopters owned by news organizations were doing what he referred to as "endless loops" around the neighborhood. Beneath their humming sounds, camera crews near a specific apartment complex tried to capture what was happening. Even before he got to work that morning, Dustin had a feeling that something was wrong. On his drive to work, for example, there were roadblocks that caused him to take a detour from his typical route. Traffic was

* This requirement partly explains why the use of these services by poor African immigrants is generally high (DeShaw 2006).

backed up on several roads close to Holly Hill, while police cars lined the roads closer to Troh's apartment. Journalists seemed to be everywhere. One was a well-known employee of CNN, who Dustin saw conducting a live report from the scene. Finally, he heard the news, and it was shocking. Someone from the neighborhood had been diagnosed with Ebola.

On another side of town, Lydia, an employee of another nonprofit organization, heard the news on the radio. While the specific details were still unclear, the news confirmed that someone in the city had been diagnosed with Ebola. Without knowing who it was, Lydia took a quick guess—that it either must be someone living in Vickery Meadow or a member of "a big fancy church" in the city who had gone on a missions trip to Africa. The more she thought about it, though, the more she believed it was the former. Over the years, the neighborhood had attracted a seemingly constant flow of new immigrants, including many people from Africa. Thus, no other neighborhood was as qualified to be ground zero of an Ebola outbreak.

From the outset of the crisis, several things were clear. America's first Ebola diagnosis was going to attract significant attention from the media, which was going to put the spotlight on Dallas residents, especially those from Africa. Additionally, the outbreak was going to be seen through a lens that connected it with neighborhood disadvantage. Whoever had the disease lived in Vickery Meadow, a neighborhood known for its poverty and blight, a place that some people referred to as the "Meadow Ghetto." It was a place so synonymous with immigrants from poor countries that Lydia had correctly guessed where the person lived just from hearing the news about the Ebola diagnosis.

Word of the diagnosis quickly reached the African community. No one had expected this to happen, but it was too soon to determine whether the infected person was really an African. Therefore, when George, an official of the CLA, learned of the first confirmed Ebola case while watching the news, he was concerned, but not as much as he was after he started receiving a flurry of calls. The calls were from members of the local media who had learned that the patient was from Liberia and wanted to talk to leaders of the community to learn more. George could not confirm that the person was from Liberia. Nevertheless, the calls kept on coming. National media outlets were also calling to talk to community leaders; however, what was happening was confusing. How had they gotten his phone number? Furthermore, at that point he simply did not have the information they were requesting. These were some of the feelings he expressed:

> The press is very interesting. I did not know they can get your contact just like that. I was at work and we were talking about [the news], and I got calls from all people from some of the major news networks. They were trying to find out who it was, but I did not know who it was at the time. I was watching TV at work, I think it was on a Monday, and that was how I learned about the first person who had entered the US with the virus. After the press called me, I was informed that it was a person from Liberia. I was told that the person was in Dallas, and they wanted to know if I knew who it was.

When he got home, the questions continued. He was shocked to find journalists waiting for him at his house and did not know how they knew where he lived. He answered their questions as politely as he could, but he still did not know who had been diagnosed. Later that evening, he learned who it was. The information came from two sources, and he described that sequence of events as follows: "And then I got a call from Liberia, from someone from one of their news agencies. He is the one who told me who it was. I don't know how he got that information. A friend of mine in the community also found out who it was and called to tell me. She had contacted me, but I did not want to disclose that information to the press."

Refusing to disclose Duncan's identity was important for several reasons. For one, it was not clear what public knowledge of his identity would imply for Liberian immigrants. Community leaders needed more time to think through these issues. No one knew how the public would react if they knew that someone with Ebola had traveled all the way from Liberia to the United States. Another reason for caution was the need to respect the patient's privacy. If reporters had been able to track George to his house, their ability to track down Duncan could not be questioned. It was also important to protect the identity of his hosts. At this point, no one knew who brought him to the country, whether they were also infected, or how they would react to all the attention.

Relentless in their bid to discover the patient's identity, journalists extended their contacts to other community leaders. One of them was Bishop Roberts, who was slightly more prepared for this than George. Earlier that morning, Roberts received a call from a contact in the community informing him of rumors that someone from Liberia had brought Ebola to the city. A few hours later, he received his first call from the media. It was from the Associated Press, and this first call was followed by calls from CNN, BBC, and VOA. In between these calls, Roberts received information from another contact in the community confirming the identity of the infected person. However, like George, he was reluctant to release the name to the media, but as he recalled, he unwittingly let it slip during a subsequent call with another media organization:

> Then one lady called me from the *Wall Street Journal*, and she said, "Bishop Roberts, we just learned that the young man's name is Thomas Duncan. Does that name sound correct?" And then I made a mistake. I said, "Yes." Next thing you know, I looked and it was already flashing on the news that "Bishop Roberts said. . ." So what I did was I called them. The local news guys here from Channel 8, I called them because they all write a lot of news articles on me, so I called them and said, "Well, there are a lot of Liberians named Thomas Duncan, so you're making [a] mistake [by not] verifying it, and saying it is Thomas Duncan. Which Thomas Duncan?"

As expected, these efforts to conceal Duncan's identity did not last long. Media organizations soon confirmed that he was indeed the person diagnosed with the disease, and that he was a guest of someone living in Vickery Meadow. With this identity confirmed, the response to the outbreak entered a new phase: a phase of intense fear. This fear was not only driven by the realization that a deadly virus now threatened the lives of Americans but also by concerns that Duncan may have started unknown chains of viral transmission within the city.

Media reports tracing Duncan's movements after his arrival from Liberia only made things worse. As Hennessey-Fiske (2014) indicates, the public wanted to know who he had been in contact with and where those people had shopped, gone to the gym, or had their nails done. Between the time of Duncan's arrival and his Ebola diagnosis, he had been in contact with close to fifty people (Weiss 2014). Approximately half of these interactions happened after he started showing symptoms, that is, around time when the virus was most contagious. Because these individuals had interacted with others in the community, the potential population at risk of infection was extensive. It included students attending two elementary schools, a middle school, and a high school in the neighborhood (Swanson et al. 2014) as well as visitors to the hospital where Duncan was admitted.

At Troh's apartment complex, residents had their own fears after hearing reports that Duncan was seen vomiting outside Troh's apartment before boarding an ambulance for the hospital (Reuters 2014a). Complicating these fears was the fact that many residents of the complex were refugees. More recent refugees, who spoke very little English, if any at all, could tell that something was wrong; however, they did not know what it was. Fearing for their lives, the few who understood English and had friends in the neighborhood left the complex to stay with those friends. As Lydia, whose organization provides services to refugees in the community, explained, refugees witnessed dramatic scenes of helicopters, journalists, and hazmat teams moving around the complex but lacked translation services to inform them of what was really happening. It was, as she put it,

> very difficult, especially at [Troh's apartment complex], because there are a lot of different languages there, and the older kids started translating for everybody, including the press, which was like, "Oh, my gosh." But some people were newly here; here I am in a foreign country and there are all these people in hazmat suits; the helicopter was over the community for [what] seemed like a month. I guess it was just a couple of weeks, but a helicopter all day every day. There were people in uniforms, people in emergency vehicles all throughout the neighborhood, what seemed like—again, I don't have a real sense of time because it seemed like it went on forever, and so they're scared to death. They didn't know what [was] going on, [and] people didn't have words [to] tell them.

Several agencies developed strategies to provide refugees with information on the outbreak and to offer other types of assistance at their offices. These agencies prepared flyers in the native languages of major refugee groups and posted them on walls in the complex. One of these efforts was led by the CDC, which sent out similar notices that were translated into Spanish, French, Vietnamese, and other major languages. However, this strategy had one limitation: it meant that refugees from smaller groups, such as those from Burma or the Congo, did not receive notices in their native language.

In some cases, the sight of the notices only served to increase refugees' fears. Some were unable to read or found it difficult to understand what was supposedly written in their language. As Lydia recalled, "[The CDC's] stuff was written in ways that people couldn't understand. . . . They had some things in different languages, but those who could speak the languages were going [laughs], 'This doesn't make sense for us.'" Consequently, refugee organizations started fielding their questions and opening their offices to those who wanted to meet with caseworkers. As Dustin explained, this was done to help those who did not know what Ebola was as well as those who wanted to know whether it was safe to go to work, send their children to school, or do things of that nature.

The Spread of Fear and the Opportunity to Blame

With the saturation of the media with news of Duncan's diagnosis, new concerns emerged among Africans about what it meant for their own lives. For Africans living in Vickery Meadow, the immediate fear was for their personal safety. Among those who expressed these fears was a group of poor African immigrant women who were served by an organization run by Negasi, who was from Ethiopia. Like other residents in Troh's apartment complex, these women were concerned about accidentally contracting the disease in the neighborhood. Furthermore, they stopped going to the THP hospital out of concern that it had been contaminated by Duncan. New fears further emerged among other African groups, especially those with links to the West African countries tied to the epidemic. Eku, for example, claimed that it was not so much the death of Duncan that concerned them but the subsequent infection of the nurses who treated him. It confirmed that the virus had started to spread. From her perspective, therefore, "it was pretty scary," especially after they "learned about the people who had treated [Duncan] and how they became sick and almost died as a result of that and all." Given that Eku had lost a cousin, who was a doctor, under similar circumstances in Sierra Leone, her concerns were not abstract. The infection of the nurses appeared to follow a pattern. It suggested that the outbreak was going to have similar consequences in Dallas as the epidemic had in West Africa.

None of these fears matched the level of concern that emerged among Liberian immigrants. After all, it was specifically this group of Africans who had interacted with Duncan the most. They included Troh and her children, guests who stopped by their house to welcome Duncan, and friends who occasionally visited Troh's family. Among the last to visit was a cousin of Paul, a community leader. In the weeks leading up to Duncan's arrival, his cousin had been a frequent guest at Troh's residence. However, shortly after Duncan's arrival he became homeless and had moved in with Paul's family while he tried to get back on his feet. As word got out that Duncan had been diagnosed with Ebola, Paul became concerned because he was aware of his cousin's relationship with Troh. When he asked his cousin whether he had recently visited Troh's apartment, he replied that he had not, but Paul subsequently found out that this was not true, and he became concerned that his family was in danger. Still bewildered as he recalled the incident, he gave the following account:

> When he was asked whether he had visited there, after Duncan's diagnosis was confirmed, he lied and said he had not visited there. Can you imagine how concerned we were in our house? Ebola could have come to our house. He lived in my house. If my cousin had Ebola. . . He had his own shower on his side of our house. But if he drank from a cup and someone else drinks from it, everyone in the house would have been contaminated. Yes, I was scared. But I asked him, "Is it true that you have been visiting there?" He lied. He said no. But people had seen him there. When he found out that Ebola was there, he stopped going there.

Other residents responded with a mixture of fear and disappointment. Assurances from officials that the healthcare system was capable of responding to the outbreak were met with skepticism. To many of them, it was these same officials who allowed someone with the disease to travel all the way from Liberia to the United States without being detected. They could not be trusted because they had failed to stop Duncan. Public distrust of the authorities was coupled with widespread ignorance about the ways in which the disease was transmitted. For example, the threat of Ebola was magnified by the belief that the virus could spread through the air or through water (Swanson et al. 2014).

Nationally, the fear of Ebola expanded as media coverage of Duncan's experiences increased. Shortly after his death, a *Washington Post*–ABC news poll revealed that more than two-thirds of Americans had fears about the possible spread of the epidemic (Dennis and Craighill 2014). As a result of these fears, some people started to travel wearing face masks, while others contributed to the rising sales of hand sanitizer (Tuttle 2014). On Wall Street, stock prices for airline companies declined as concerns about the effects of the virus on the traveling industry increased. Part of the hysteria was driven by the media's quest to track down the movements of those who had been infected (Monson 2017). For example, fears about the safety of air travel were triggered by news reports that Amber Vinson had traveled on a commercial airliner the day before she started showing symptoms (Garza and Wade 2014). Similar fears were expressed by employees of the airline industry itself. In New York, for example, cabin cleaners employed by an airline company refused to work out of fear that they were insufficiently protected (Gambino 2014a).

Soon people feared that they could contract Ebola from anyone or anything associated with the city of Dallas. In Maine, a teacher at Strong Elementary School was placed on a twenty-one-day leave after returning from a conference held ten miles from the THP hospital (Byrne 2014). Additionally, plans to dispose of the ash derived from the incineration of linens, bedding, and carpet taken from Troh's apartment were halted. The receiving facility at Lake Charles, Louisiana, refused to accept it until they were sure it posed no risk to the health of their community (Dallas News Administrator 2014).

As the search for explanations to understand these fears began, the social response shifted to the development of a narrative of blame. At this point, the focus of the narrative was on Duncan, and its main objective was to understand the extent to which his actions or his social characteristics played a role in making him the focus of the crisis. However, unlike previous accounts that focus on how immigrants are blamed during epidemics (Markel and Stern 2002; Nelkin and Gilman 1988), the evolving narrative had two origins. One came from individuals outside the African immigrant community and the other from African immigrants themselves.

Outside the community, the most common narrative of blame was one that placed disproportionate responsibility for the outbreak on the actions of Duncan. This narrative was advanced from several directions. The first was based on his apparent deception. It maintained that he knew exactly what he was doing, and that he deliberately traveled to the United States because he did not stand a chance of surviving in Liberia after becoming infected. Thus, he was blamed for failing to tell authorities at the airport in

Monrovia that he had been in contact with someone who was infected with the virus (Onishi and Santora 2014). The second narrative, related to the first, focused on Duncan's perceived irresponsibility. Accordingly, he was blamed for not telling the nurses at the THP hospital that he had recently been in contact with someone who was sick or had Ebola (Balluck 2014). However, this claim was disputed by his fiancée, who maintained that Duncan could not have known that the pregnant woman he assisted in Liberia had been infected with the virus (Troh 2015).

Within the African community, however, the search for explanations began with a rejection of this outside narrative. This response was based on the belief that Duncan was unfairly faulted for causing the outbreak, and that his experience was the outcome of systemic failures that occurred both in the United States and in Liberia. To make this point clear, some Liberians made a clear distinction between the circumstances of Duncan's travel to the United States and those of Patrick Sawyer. The latter was the Liberian American national who was infected with Ebola and is believed to have deliberately traveled from Liberia to Nigeria to seek care earlier in the epidemic. Liberians argued that, unlike Duncan, Sawyer not only knew that his sister had been infected with Ebola, but he had also been observed to be sick while at the airport. In Duncan's case, the facts were not so clear. He left Liberia as all travelers did during that time, that is, after successfully passing the screening tests at the airport. While Sawyer's decision to leave Liberia was thought to be planned, Duncan's was seen as serendipitous. In other words, it was seen to have helped place him in the United States before he knew he was infected, and in so doing it put him in a context where he was more likely to get advanced medical attention. In fact, there was some sense that Duncan's ordeal was an opportune moment in the crisis because it forced the world to pay attention to the epidemic in Africa at a time when few people were taking it seriously.

Rather than blame Duncan for the outbreak in the city, many Africans chose to focus on the hospital and its employees as the main cause of the crisis. Accordingly, when Tayo, a community leader from Sierra Leone, heard about the Ebola case in the city, he was shocked. He first learned about it during a call he received from a reporter asking him to comment on the diagnosis. Subsequently, his shock gave way to anger as he attempted to understand why a leading hospital in the city had initially failed to correctly diagnose the cause of Duncan's illness. As he described it: "I was a little ticked off by the fact that he came down with this thing, [and] they sent him home. It wasn't like they had never heard about this thing and that people did not think it was going to come here. They'd been talking and being suspicious about that, and were saying 'We are ready,' 'We are ready,' and then they happen to send him home? Luckily, he didn't spread it to 1,500 people."

Race, Ethnicity, and Blame for the Outbreak

Even more central to the narrative of blame that was developed within the African immigrant community were explanations focusing on the role of racial disadvantage. They not only served to contest the narrative of Duncan's deception but also provided an opportunity for African Americans to participate in the emerging discourse on the crisis. The racial narrative also allowed many Africans to link Duncan's experiences with discrimination to their own. This narrative sought to answer whether Duncan's predicament reflected the Black racial disadvantage typically observed in the provision of healthcare services and interrogated the larger social context in which his experiences occurred. Much of the concern about the racial undertones of the crisis focused on the former. Indeed, the question of whether Duncan's fate was determined by his race was at the heart of a national debate. Raising the possibility that his death was explained by racism, for example, Ellison (2014) rhetorically questions how one of the best-equipped hospitals in Dallas could send a West African patient home after he complained that he was sick. Others pushed back at this notion of racism, with one individual calling it an unproductive diversion. Instead, they argued that what had occurred was a consequence of other factors, such as human error.

As with this broader debate, the issue of racial discrimination was far from settled among Africans in the city, and their perspectives straddled both sides of the debate. The popular view was that he would have received much better care at the hospital had he been a White American. Others simply questioned why he was not offered ZMapp, the same experimental drug given to Brantly and Writebol, who recovered from the disease. Some saw this as evidence of discrimination, while others seemed content with simply highlighting the disparity. Troh, for example, was befuddled as to why the drug had not been offered to Duncan; instead, after his condition advanced from serious to critical, he was offered a less effective experimental drug called Brincidofovir, which was originally developed to treat smallpox and adenovirus (Jacobson 2014).*

Although Troh's main concern was about the effectiveness of the treatment, her specific views on the role of race in the care Duncan received are a useful starting point in examining the discrimination perspective. Grounding her views in what she saw while they were at the hospital, Troh dismissed the notion that Duncan was a victim of racial prejudice. Indeed, she did not view the decision of the first doctors who sent him home during their initial visit to be a result of racial prejudice. Speaking of the doctor, she said: "Was he treating us less than others because we were Black? Because we were foreigners? I do not think so. If I saw that I would have complained" (Troh 2015, 123). At the same time, she did not discount the possibility that Duncan's overall experience was negatively affected by other types of barriers. Thus, she speculated that a second factor, citizenship status, would have made all the difference in terms of the level of care he received. "Maybe," she surmised, "if Eric [i.e., Thomas] had been a citizen, that doctor would have wanted to help him more" (Troh 2015, 123).

Africans in the city who believed Duncan was a victim of racism were less speculative as they affirmed their convictions on what happened. To them, Duncan simply died because he was Black. This notion was particularly salient among working-class immigrants, who offered intuitive arguments to justify their conclusions. The most obvious was based on a juxtaposition of the racial characteristics of Duncan and those of the two Ebola-infected Americans evacuated from Liberia. As such, the fact that these White Americans received more favorable treatment and survived while Duncan did not was taken as evidence to conclude that he was a victim of racial discrimination. This was what Saran, an immigrant from Ivory Coast, was referring to when she raised the following questions at a hair-braiding salon she was visiting: "First of all, why did they leave the guy to die? That was a big question on the minds of everyone, because

---

* It was thought that the drug would also help people infected with Ebola, but it failed to improve Duncan's prognosis. Kent Brantly also offered to donate blood to Duncan because doctors believed that the plasma of Ebola survivors contained antibodies that could help infected persons recover from the virus. However, his blood type did not match Duncan's.

those people who got infected, those White people, they got healed, right? So why did this African, we have to add the word 'African' . . . yeah, why did they let him die? [Brantly and Writebol] came straight over here and got healed, so why is it that [Duncan], who also got infected over there, died after he came here? Big question mark."

While Saran was a student living close to Vickery Meadow, she was no stranger to Ebola. She first heard about the virus while living in her native Ivory Coast, a country where Ebola outbreaks had occurred in the past. As a result, she knew that the chances of recovering from the disease were slim. However, her faith in the ability of Americans to cure the disease had increased when both Dr. Kent Brantly and Nancy Writebol recovered after they were brought back to the United States. Given these events, therefore, it did not make sense to her that Duncan, who was infected in the same country and who just happened to be Black, died while they survived.

Saran was convinced that the source of the problem was the THP hospital. She went on to say that because of her fears and concerns, she would no longer visit the THP hospital when she was sick. She was concerned that if the hospital had allowed Duncan to die because he was a Black African, it would do the same to her. Thus, she concluded: "If I go there, they could kill me because I'm African. . . . If they let an African die, if they see my card and see that I am not American—I'm 100 percent African—even if they hear my accent, I'm dead."

To Saran, therefore, Duncan's fate was the outcome of a specific type of racial disadvantage—that faced by Black Africans like herself. This was a nuanced perspective that combined the conventional notion of anti-Black racism with that of an African ethnic disadvantage. In the past, it has been used to advance the argument for a more intense level of prejudice experienced by African immigrants (Dodoo 1997). In part, this ethnoracial disadvantage is believed to be influenced by negative stereotypes about Africa held by Americans, an idea that was fleshed out by Onike, an immigrant from Nigeria who worked at the salon Saran was visiting. Like Saran, she was convinced that Duncan was allowed to die; however, she saw this as part of a larger effort to promote the notion that Ebola was an African disease. In order to make her point, she attempted to make connections between Duncan's death and stereotypical views of Africans she had seen on TV: "[The media] made it look like [Ebola] was an African thing. I remember I was watching TV one day. . . . I was so mad when they said that in Grand Prairie, they had an African killer bee [laughs]. So in my mind, I was thinking, 'How did a bee fly all the way from Africa to Grand Prairie?' And they named it 'killer' bee, so an American bee doesn't kill? But African bee—you know, it's just so much, but I mean, we're in their country, [so] we have to deal with it."

Beke, another immigrant from Nigeria, did not wait until Duncan's death to develop concerns about how his race and ethnicity could shape the type of treatment he would receive. According to her, as soon as she learned that the infected person was from Liberia, she immediately predicted that he would be allowed to die. This prediction was startling, but it was based on her perception of what Americans thought of Africans. From her perspective, Duncan's fate was settled "from the get-go . . . because he was an African," and because Americans do not really value the lives of Africans. Despite this prediction, she was still stunned by the contrast between Duncan's experiences and those of the two infected nurses who survived. Still angry as she recalled her reaction at the time, she said: "When he passed, those two nurses that got it from him were transported to, was it New York? That was what pissed me [off] the most. I [told my coworkers], 'Do you all remember what I was telling you guys? Exactly.' They did this because our lives do not really mean anything to them. You understand?"

Nevertheless, it was not just the death of Duncan that was seen to reflect these biases against Africans. They were seen in the way he was treated on the way to the hospital and in the substandard treatments he received. They were seen in the greater compassion showed to the sick nurses and in the apparently unexplained events that followed his death at the hospital. Some of these biases were captured in a statement released by Duncan's exasperated nephew following his death. He bemoaned the fact that Duncan was forced to walk from the ambulance to the THP hospital during his second visit, while the Ebola-infected Americans were carried into the hospital on stretchers. He did not understand why his family was told that Duncan's Ebola tests would take about three to seven days to come back, while the results for an officer in Texas suspected of having the virus took less than twenty-four hours (Weeks 2014). He also wondered why the two Americans infected in Liberia began their treatment with ZMapp while in Africa, but it took about nine days for Duncan's family to receive a request for consent for him to receive an experimental drug (Weeks 2014). He found this difference puzzling because, as he explained, the two Americans received their treatment while *in Africa*, while Duncan had no access to the treatment, even though he was already *in the United States* (Gambino 2014b).

With regard to differences in the level of compassion showed to Ebola-infected patients, the focus was on the contrast between public reactions to the diagnosis of Duncan and the diagnosis of Nina Pham. Compared to Duncan, who was blamed for starting the crisis, Pham received a level of sympathy that was so widespread that it was extended to her dog. She owned a Cavalier King Charles Spaniel that was initially suspected of having contracted the virus (Ayala and Rajwani 2014). During this period, concerns about its welfare were expressed in the media, during news conferences, and by people who wanted to know how it was doing. Subsequently, the media reported that the dog was Ebola-free, and that it was receiving what was referred to as royal treatment from Dallas Animal Services; the organization had vowed to do all they could to attend to its needs and return it to its owner (Wilonsky 2014). To some African immigrants, these concerns were shocking. It was not clear, according to one, why "the dog got more attention than Duncan." This perception of greater public sympathy for the dog than for Duncan was hard for them to dismiss and only served to underscore the notion that the lives of Africans were not valued.

Others were concerned with the perceived bias in the way the hospital treated Troh and her children while Duncan was admitted. It did not make sense that they were not allowed to visit him while he was in isolation, and that the hospital took no steps to make this possible. Keeping them separated was seen as a violation of African cultural norms that required one to be with their loved ones before their death and for those loved ones to provide them with their last wishes, if possible. Beke, therefore, argued that despite the fact that Ebola is infectious, the hospital should have provided personal protective equipment for Troh and her family to allow them to make some physical contact with Duncan before his death. These perceived biases became more magnified after Duncan succumbed to the disease, and part of this stemmed from the belief that his body was cremated without his family's permission. No one from the family was allowed to witness the cremation. To some, this made it difficult to confirm that Duncan had indeed been cremated, or to check for signs of physical abuse on the body before it was disposed of.

The many unknowns about what happened to Duncan's body helped to fuel conspiracy theories that constructed his ordeal as part of a plan to exploit African lives for the benefit of science. These theories were similar to those developed by Africans who questioned the origins of the Ebola virus at the start of the epidemic, in the sense that they viewed the events surrounding Duncan's death as consequences of the actions of US scientists. In this case, however, the conspiracy was not so much based on whether the virus had man-made origins but on whether Duncan's time at the hospital was used to perform medical experiments. These arguments were sometimes made in isolation, but at times they were developed in ways that incorporated the role race had in explaining the apparent mystery surrounding the way in which the corpse was disposed of.

Surprisingly, one proponent of this view was Brise, an immigrant from Cameroon with a doctoral degree from an American institution. He bought into this notion while listening to a pundit on TV discussing Duncan's case after his diagnosis was confirmed. As Brise recalled, the pundit indicated that now that the cause of Duncan's illness had been confirmed, "we are going to know everything about Ebola through this guy." He took this to mean that scientists were going to allow Duncan to go through the process of dying from the virus to help them understand how humans with Ebola died of the disease. In other words, Duncan's death was fixed. It was a planned outcome in which, according to Brise, "[scientists] saw the stages of it little by little . . . because they wanted to see him go little by little and die, and then they [would] know how somebody dies [from] Ebola. Then they'll do an autopsy and find out all that's going on, but if they treated him, he will be on the street, and they won't know exactly what happened. Here in the United States, I mean, maybe they do it out there in Africa and stuff, but here in the United States they made him die right there in front of them."

Brise further provided an important nuance to his claims of a racial conspiracy. Duncan, he argued, was exploited not just because he was a Black African but because he was seen as being untruthful. That is, the belief that he was dishonest about his prior interactions with an infected person reinforced the perception of the inferiority of his race. At this point, according to Brise, it was easy to justify using him as a candidate for conducting experiments: "In this case," he concluded, "a Black life did not matter."

Such extreme views were not held by everyone who used race to construct a narrative of blame. For many, a case for racial prejudice could still be made from a social justice perspective. In the absence of comprehensive information on why Duncan fared much worse than the other patients, the social context of racial inequality remained relevant for making sense of his experiences. This logic of incorporating the broader influence of anti-Black prejudice was also shared by others outside the African community. In one notable case, Reverend Jesse Jackson questioned why Duncan did not receive the same treatment that was given to Brantly and Writebol; moreover, he identified several social markers of disadvantage, including his race, nationality, and accent, as factors that robbed him of the opportunity to receive equal treatment (Kim and Jackson 2014). Similar concerns were also expressed in Liberia by locals who were familiar with the exceptional treatment given to Brantly and Writebol at the ELWA hospital. Duncan's death, one argued, was a consequence of American racism and xenophobia, as well as a strategy for discouraging infected Africans from seeking treatment for Ebola abroad (Hersher 2014).

As various aspects of the racial narrative gained momentum, officials pushed back by offering a nonracial alternative. This alternative emphasized the limits of diagnostic procedures used at the THP hospital, human failings, and other related factors. However, officials were not alone in advancing explanations that looked beyond race. They were joined by a number of middle-class Africans who rejected racial interpretations of Duncan's ordeal in favor of nonracial alternatives. At the core of this counternarrative were two arguments. The first was that the Duncan tragedy was not predictable, and as a result, very little could have been done to prevent it. The second argument viewed the ordeal as a consequence of a lack of planning. It maintained that despite the fact that health officials were aware of the raging epidemic in West Africa, they did very little to prepare for an outbreak in America's major cities.

By far the most common of these two ideas was the former. It was the one offered by Tayo, who refused to see the circumstances surrounding

Duncan's death through the lens of race. He was a very successful businessman from Sierra Leone and was no stranger to the THP hospital. He had used their services during the birth of his child, and his wife was a previous employee of the hospital. While recognizing the pernicious effects of racism on the lives of Africans in the city, he refused to conclude that it was the key factor that determined Duncan's fate. He explained his views as follows: "I tried again not to put everything in black and white. People make mistakes. It could have been just an honest mistake—that's what I know. It's a good hospital, has been a reputable one. My child who is now in college was born there. My wife used to work there, so it's a good hospital. I don't have anything against them. As far as whether it's discriminatory, I don't think so. I don't think so. It's one of those accidents that happen."

In the same vein, Hassan, a Sierra Leonean who worked at a university close to the city, rejected the racial nexus in favor of the narrative of inadvertency. Racism, he maintained, does matter to the extent that there was a double standard in America that is the lived reality for immigrants in the city, but, in this case, he argued, the focus on racial victimhood is incorrect. What transpired at the hospital, in his view, was simply a tragic event. It was driven by operational lapses tied to hospital workers' ignorance about the virus. As he further explained, "But in defense of [the THP hospital], they were just not familiar with the Ebola [virus] or how to react to it. Texas is not like Washington, DC, or New York City in terms of [being] a place that is cosmopolitan enough [that] you have a significant African minority that's been there for a while, so when events like this Duncan case occur, you'd have people who would empathize [with the racism view]. That was not the case here."

Conversely, Liberian community leaders focused on a nonracial narrative that was based on systemic failures that happened as a result of a lack of planning for the outbreak. As such, when Bishop Roberts discussed the lapses that occurred in Duncan's treatment, he was careful to emphasize that what happened was a product of inadequate preparation. "No one was prepared," he argued. "Nobody, not even Obama, was prepared." From this perspective, this lack of planning explained why doctors failed to test for Ebola during Duncan's first visit to the hospital. At the same time, the bishop was emphatic that Duncan's experience had no racial undertones.

Ebola, he maintained, "does not know color, so we have to stop playing the color game."

George, an official of the CLA, extended this line of thought by focusing on what occurred outside of Dallas. Like Bishop Roberts, he refused to empathize with popular claims of racism; instead, he believed that there was enough blame to go around. Liberian officials, he argued, could be blamed for the poor screening process used at the airport in Monrovia that failed to show that Duncan was infected with Ebola. If the virus had been identified at the airport in Monrovia, Duncan would not have died in Dallas, and to George this was more important than focusing on race to explain the cause of the outbreak in Dallas.

As Yomi, a Nigerian immigrant living in the community, explained, the issue of a lack of planning had an important consequence: ignorance about the signs of Ebola. It was also difficult for him to accept the notion that Duncan was a victim of racism because it was inconsistent with what he perceived to be the generosity of the US healthcare system. He did not believe that a system set up to extend services to vulnerable people during emergencies could at the same time be racist toward its patients. Thus, the only other alternative way of explaining what happened was that hospital workers simply did not know how to treat someone with Ebola. Consequently, he argued, "For what I know of America, I'll give them the benefit of [the] doubt. Whenever somebody is sick, let's say you have an accident on the road, they will take care of you in spite of who you are. I will be violating my conscience if I think they probably would have done it because of race. I think that when there was the outbreak, they did not know how to handle it. They did not know how to handle it."

Finally, one of the more intuitive explanations offered to dispel claims of racism at the THP hospital was offered by Abu, a Sierra Leonean living in Dallas. It encompassed two arguments. The first focused on changes in the physical environment around the time of Duncan's arrival in Dallas. This perspective maintained that the health changes that usually follow the transition from summer to fall possibly explained why his symptoms were initially misdiagnosed. That is, Duncan visited the hospital at the start of flu season, and many of the symptoms he reported, including fatigue and headaches, were similar to those of flu patients visiting the hospital at that time of year. Abu's second argument was that the transmission of the virus from Duncan to the nurses was itself an indication that he was not being ignored because of racism. At the very least, he maintained, the spread of the virus from Duncan to the nurses indicated that they touched him and that his vital signs were taken, things that would not have occurred if he were not given the necessary attention.

In general, therefore, there was no consensus among Africans on whether the unfortunate fate of Duncan could be blamed on racism. Claims of racial prejudice were countered with arguments that rejected its influence as an explanation for the outbreak. The rejection of the racial narrative was carefully done in a way that focused on the specific experiences of Duncan; it was not a complete denial of its broader social significance. However, individuals on both sides of the debate failed to recognize that their main arguments were not mutually exclusive. Neither the argument of inadvertency nor that of inadequate planning precludes exposure to racial biases in the healthcare system. Likewise, the transmission of the virus from Duncan to the two nurses could have occurred even if the initial misdiagnosis of his condition was a consequence of racial prejudice. African immigrants' views on the importance of racism were nevertheless important insofar as they tell us what they considered to be the major causes of the outbreak in the city. Still, they tell us very little about the significance of another factor, that is, access to health insurance, as an additional explanation for why the outbreak occurred.

Access to Health Insurance and the Dallas Ebola Crisis

The challenge of access to health insurance was more than just an idea developed to promote an alternative narrative for understanding Duncan's ordeal. Within the African community, it was part of life and was particularly important for two major groups of people: those in low-income families and recently arrived immigrants. Refugees were partly protected from these challenges because they received support through Medicaid for about six months after they arrived in the United States. Before the end of this period, refugees are expected to find jobs that will provide them with health insurance, but this is not always possible. The challenge associated with access to health insurance was also faced by entrepreneurs in the community. They were not always able to afford the high premiums required by local insurance providers and still be able to make a profit.

Some community leaders believed that the broader problem of access to health insurance was made worse by cultural factors. Most African immigrants arrived from countries where national health insurance services were unavailable. At the time of the Ebola epidemic in Liberia, for example, the country did not have a national health insurance system. Instead, the most reliable services available were offered in the private sector, which covered only about 15 percent of the population (Josephson et al. 2014).

Undocumented immigrant status also posed a barrier to accessing health insurance in the city because it limits immigrants' access to the kinds of jobs that offer health insurance benefits. After Congress passed the Affordable Care Act in 2010, many immigrants were able to benefit from the subsidies provided by the program. However, in order to receive these benefits, they needed to either be naturalized US citizens or permanent residents who had been residing in the United States for at least five years (Joseph 2016). However, even these groups of eligible immigrants included low-income families who struggled to make other out-of-pocket payments for healthcare.

Onike put these constraints into context when she discussed how Duncan could have been disadvantaged otherwise. She indicated that she worked as a hair-braider because she was unable to find a job that allowed her to use the public administration degree she earned in Nigeria. Influenced by her own experience in seeking care at the THP hospital, she lamented how difficult it was to receive treatment without health insurance. After she found out that she needed to have a minor procedure, she was told by a THP hospital employee that because she lacked health insurance, she needed to pay $4,800 up front in order to get it done. She could not afford it, so she chose to wait it out. Based on this experience, she believed that in addition to experiencing racial discrimination, Duncan also received substandard treatment from the THP hospital, especially during his first visit, because he had no access to health insurance.

Duncan's vulnerability reflected the fact that he epitomized some of the major risk factors associated with limited access to health insurance in the community. He was from a low-income group, which meant that he would not have been able to afford private travel insurance before leaving Liberia. Moreover, although he legally traveled to the United States, he was neither a legal permanent resident nor a naturalized US citizen. Given that he was in the country visiting his family, he also would not have qualified for sub-sidies provided by social programs such as Medicare. Because of this, many Africans believed that Duncan's experience could also be blamed on bar-riers created by the lack of health insurance.

Community members used two perspectives to advance this notion. The first focused on the ways in which the lack of health insurance stig-matized Duncan as a financial burden to the hospital. As someone who owns a business that provides healthcare services, Tayo was one of those convinced that the hospital sent Duncan home during his first visit be-cause of his lack of health insurance. This possibility, he claimed, was more likely than the notion that the decision was based on his race. To make his argument, Tayo began by observing a notable shift that occurred in the insurance market after the passing of the Affordable Care Act. While the act had made it easier for poor people to get access to healthcare, he ar-gued, patients without health insurance have been increasingly seen as a burden because it is difficult to be reimbursed for services provided to them. Thus, he maintained, "the insurance issue had a part to play in how Duncan was treated. They knew he did not have insurance, so they did not want to spend more than they needed to, so they just gave him Tylenol and whatever they wanted to give him and sent him home. It's a possibil-ity. It happens a lot of times."

Eku, who similarly disagreed with the racial prejudice hypothesis, clar-ified the issue further. What occurred during Duncan's first visit, she be-lieved, was consistent with what healthcare institutions do to meet the basic requirements of the law. In other words, she continued, because they are required to treat all patients during emergencies regardless of their ability to pay, the hospital very likely focused on treating Duncan's symp-toms rather than conducting a thorough diagnosis.* Eku further reasoned that the insurance angle could not be dismissed because one of the first questions asked to patients after they arrive at a hospital is whether they have health insurance. It was at that point, she believed, that Duncan's neg-ative response to the question influenced how he was subsequently treated.

---

* Other accounts dispute this reasoning and indicate that Duncan was tested for a num-ber of ailments, including stroke and appendicitis, during his first visit to the hospital (Gam-bino 2014b).

The second perspective was based not so much on how the lack of health insurance affected the THP hospital's response but on the fact that, as an institution that served patients with high rates of insurance, it had no experience treating populations with no health insurance. Most poor immigrants in the community who did not have health insurance visited FQHCs such as the Parkland County hospital rather than the THP hospital. This difference had a number of implications. For example, many believed that FQHCs would not have turned Duncan away nor would they have conducted a less thorough diagnosis of his ailment because he lacked health insurance. More importantly, most immigrants who visit FQHCs close to Vickery Meadow are from the developing world. As such, there was a perception that doctors at these centers would have been better able to diagnose an Ebola infection correctly because of their vast expertise in dealing with tropical diseases.

One person who had this view was Nancy, a trained nurse. As she explained, these issues are not just theoretical but reflected the realities of her job. She began by setting the context to show how patients of the county hospital where she worked are different: "We have patients literally from all countries of the world, literally, and a lot of the immigrants come from, of course, West Africa. Then you have the Caribbean, South America, Mexico and Guatemala, Honduras, those countries, and we have lots of Africans from all over Africa, Kenyans and all that. So I said, 'Oh, well, maybe this is [Duncan's] opportunity to get treated.'" Next, she focused on why the distinction between county hospitals and the THP hospital could have made the difference in Duncan's outcome. In the process, she underscored the importance of the main distinctions that mattered—county hospitals' limited concern about patients' ability to pay and their vigilance in preparing for viruses such as Ebola. "Unfortunately, I always say that if that patient—and this is my personal feeling because I work in a county hospital—had not gone to a private hospital like Presbyterian, I feel like he may have survived. I believe that county hospitals, because we have so many patients from across the globe and because we don't look at patients based on their ability to pay but treat them no matter what, are usually more vigilant with things like this. . . . I believe that, probably, the outcome would have been different."

The notion that the THP hospital was a poor fit for Duncan's ailment was not just held by Nancy but by others outside the African community. Brady, an American healthcare professional at a county hospital in the city, made a slightly similar argument. Unlike Nancy, he was not sure that the difference was in how the THP hospital treated patients without insurance. Instead, the main issue, he believed, was that the THP hospital simply did not have enough experience working with ethnically diverse immigrants. This point was important because the hospital is located close to Vickery Meadow and occasionally treated immigrants from the neighborhood. However, compared to poor immigrants, the majority of its clients were privileged. They were members of the city's middle class and upper class—people who appreciated the sophisticated music played at the baby grand piano on the hospital's second floor. Thus, as Brady implied, there was a sharp social disconnect between the THP hospital and the poor residents of Vickery Meadow, who lived within walking distance. Because of these differences, he concluded, when an immigrant patient with Duncan's symptoms shows up on their doorstep, "somebody working at that hospital, even the ER, would not necessarily think of a third world illness. They won't put two and two together."

All told, explanations that focused on the lack of health insurance were used as part of a larger narrative developed to shift the blame from Duncan toward other factors perceived to be responsible for the crisis. As shown earlier in the chapter, this metanarrative consisted of loosely connected subnarratives that focused on how racial and nonracial factors shaped the origins of the outbreak. Despite disagreement among Africans about which of these was the most important, one thing was clear. At the core of each narrative is the realization that Duncan's death was partly a consequence of his low social and economic status and partly a consequence of health system failures. In this sense, they all agreed that Duncan's death did not have to happen. It could have been prevented under a different set of circumstances.

The Dallas Ebola Crisis in Perspective

We cannot discount the fact that news of the first case of Ebola diagnosed in the United States helped raise public awareness of an ongoing epidemic in West Africa. However, this awareness had several consequences for the lives of Americans and Africans living in Dallas. It caused many

Americans to experience feelings of vulnerability to circumstances that were beyond their control. Added to this, it caused them to confront a new set of conditions that required them to react to a direct threat to their lives. Many of these feelings were also felt by Africans in the city. But for those from the West African countries directly affected by the virus, the outbreak marked a unique phase in their experience—one that required them to balance their concerns about the spreading virus in Africa with the immediate realities of its consequences in their neighborhoods.

While the specific implications of the outbreak differed for various groups, they were all united in their initial response to the crisis. Realizing that prior assurances that healthcare institutions were prepared for an outbreak had failed, the first set of responses were those based on expressions of fear. Subsequently, in the absence of credible answers to explain what had just happened, an emerging narrative of blame was used to make sense of the causes of the crisis. At this point, it focused exclusively on the fate of Duncan. Outside the African community, the emerging narrative advanced the notion that Duncan knew he was infected before leaving Liberia and lied to get access to healthcare services. Within the community, however, this narrative was largely rejected. In its place, African immigrants developed their own metanarrative of blame in order to come to terms with what occurred at the THP hospital.

How these immigrants interpreted this was a different matter. There were notable variations in their understanding of these events that formed the basis of several subnarratives. The most common was focused on arguments of racial prejudice and was based on their subjective perceptions of racism. But while this argument was subjective, it was consistent with the large body of evidence on racial and ethnic inequalities in how patients are treated in the healthcare system (Feagin and Bennefield 2014; Harris et al. 1997; Klabunde et al. 1998). The subnarrative on the lack of planning was also compelling, and it enabled immigrants to correctly argue that the initial misdiagnosis of Duncan would not have occurred had the THP hospital been more prepared for an outbreak. Finally, the subnarrative on constraints associated with access to health insurance was important for highlighting the direct and indirect ways in which Duncan was disadvantaged. As with the racial narrative, it matched the realities of many in the community and was widely recognized as a barrier limiting their access to healthcare.

Each of the subnarratives represents important claims that cannot be ignored, and the validity of one does not undermine the validity of another. At the same time, they are instructive for recognizing the fact that during Duncan's first encounter with a US hospital, he faced a combination of social disadvantages that were not experienced by any Ebola-infected American during the epidemic. Although competing claims of Duncan's deception were also important, they were less rooted in fact compared to claims of the lack of health insurance or the inadequate planning for the outbreak. Ultimately, therefore, it is these factors that are perhaps the most important for understanding the social origins of the crisis in Dallas.

This does not imply that perceptions of the influence of race and ethnicity on Duncan's experiences were not important. They certainly were. And as I will demonstrate shortly, race and ethnicity became considerably more important for understanding the responses observed during the next phase of the outbreak. Soon after coming to terms with the start of the crisis, the attention of the public shifted from Duncan to groups perceived to pose a similar threat. This shift led to a major transformation in the narrative of blame, from the focus on one individual to groups with similar racial and ethnic characteristics. What this shift implied for life among Africans in the city was significant. The crisis was about to have collective consequences for the African community that were observed on a scale that had never been seen before.

6 Africans as Untouchables

Vickery Meadow seemed like a great place for Kiragu to start his small-scale humanitarian project. After arriving in the United States from Kenya, he had experienced some measure of success running his own business in Dallas, and as a result he developed the project as a way of giving back to the community. The project itself was very modest. Early each fall, he set up a booth at the apartment complex where Troh lived and handed out small gifts to the refugee residents. It was a small gesture, and the gifts were nothing fancy—bottled water and a small range of personal hygiene products. The refugees frequently stopped by to receive them from Kiragu, after which they expressed their thanks. Occasionally, he was joined in this exercise by his friend Kosmas, who was also from Kenya. While many people in Dallas avoided the neighborhood in the weeks following Duncan's death, Kiragu and Kosmas decided to continue their tradition of helping the people of Vickery Meadow. This time, however, the reception they received was different. Although the refugees were still around, they stopped coming by to receive the gifts being offered to them. Kiragu was shocked, but he knew what had happened. "The people knew we were African," he reasoned. "Nobody was greeting us anymore, nobody wanted to talk, [and] people were like, 'The water you are freely giving to us, absolutely take it back.'"

To these refugees, what seemed to matter was the apparent connection between the Ebola virus and Africans. This connection was at the heart of the stigma of Ebola that was experienced not just by the two Kenyans but by other Africans as well. It was also seen in social interactions among refugee groups within the complex. According to Kiragu, there were three groups of African refugees living in the complex at the time—refugees from

Liberia, Somalia, and Burundi—with the rest being mainly from Asia. Following the death of Duncan, there was a distinct pattern of changes in the interactions among these groups, changes that caused Africans like Kiragu to be systematically ostracized. It was a pattern that led Kiragu to draw a remarkable conclusion: "Nobody wanted to get close to African people [because] Africans were kind of untouchables." In other words, they were untouchable in the sense that they were like the Dalit groups in India. These groups, who are also referred to as untouchables, have a distinct lower caste status that subjects them to systematic patterns of discrimination and exclusion (Ram 2004).

Social relations between Africans and the rest of the Dallas public were defined by similar experiences of stigma after the start of the Ebola outbreak. As these immigrants experienced this stigma, it was clear that they were being targeted for their perceived association with Duncan. The stigma they encountered was systematic; it was linked with processes of labeling and stereotyping, as well as the use of degrading metaphors to describe Africans in terms that obscured their sense of humanity. After Duncan became sick, for example, there were calls for people who were diagnosed with Ebola in the United States to be "put down humanely" (Troh 2015, 222).* The subsequent backlash morphed into the use of more disturbing rhetoric, including a suggestion for a nuclear bomb to be dropped on Liberia as a way of controlling the growing epidemic (Cassidy 2014).

In Dallas, the embodiment of the threat of Ebola quickly extended beyond Duncan to anything associated with him. This included specific places, such as the apartment complex where he lived, and specific groups of people, including anyone who fit the profile of an African. Perceptions of the latter were broadly defined. Accordingly, although Duncan was most closely associated with the Liberian population in the city, public perception of the threat of Ebola was too unsophisticated to properly distinguish Liberians from other Africans. Identifying the threat of Ebola required people

* This was one of the more extreme examples. It was found in a tweet about Thomas Duncan and sent out by a lawyer in South Carolina indicating that "people with Ebola in the US needed to be humanely put down immediately" (Troh 2015, 222). Troh used the tweet to argue that the backlash against Duncan was so extensive that some people treated him worse than they did their animals (Troh 2015).

to make quick judgments. Such judgments necessitated the use of a reductionist strategy that made it easy to tie the risk of infection to markers, such as Africanness, that should be avoided.

Experiences of stigma observed during the Ebola crisis are important for developing an accurate portrait of the social implications of epidemics. In the case of Africans in Dallas, this stage of the epidemic was defined by several characteristics. It involved the saturation of the fear of the virus as well as the development of a clear narrative to justify the deployment of stigma. Drawing from negative stereotypes of African heritage, the main feature of this narrative was the racialization of African immigrants as being inherently different. It was thus a narrative that specifically focused on Black Africans in order to increase its appeal in a social context stratified by race. This focus had several consequences, one of which was to direct public attention toward communities associated with Duncan and not toward those associated with the other Ebola-infected persons in the city.

This stage of the epidemic also involved incorporating a reductionist perspective of Africa into a related narrative of blame. Skewed perceptions of Africans as members of a single racialized outgroup were important for developing the ideological rationale for marginalizing members of their community. This reductionist perspective was important in terms of its similarity to historical strategies used to define Africanness in terms of primitive societies. Some of the oldest attempts to frame perceptions of African identity in the West were those developed by Europeans who linked Africa with savagery, backwardness, and racial inferiority during their first series of contact with the continent (Jordan 2012). These negative stereotypes about Africa have become so globalized that it is now easy to use them in the stigmatization of Africans in countries other than the United States. However, in all these contexts the stigma of Ebola was associated with fear-based narratives that linked Africans with stereotypes that saw them as endowed with attributes that were tainted (Goffman 1963).

Nevertheless, we cannot understand these processes of stigma without acknowledging the diverse set of actors that were involved in the process of marginalizing individuals in the African immigrant community. Indeed, it was not just members of the public who were participating in the process of ostracizing these immigrants. Another set of actors were African immigrants who deployed secondary patterns of stigma toward perceived threats of the virus within their communities. Examining the role of these actors requires a recognition of the complex pathways through which stigma is deployed. The typical pathway involves less socially powerful groups, such as African immigrants, being the targets of stigma, while more powerful groups are the sources of stigma. Yet, the outbreak in Dallas was different. In the context of extreme fear of Ebola and the presence of Africans from diverse national groups, many opportunities were available for observing additional pathways of stigma.

These disease-related stigmas have real consequences for the well-being of stigmatized persons, and there is no shortage of studies reporting the negative effects of the stigma of Ebola during the epidemic. In West Africa, for example, these effects were observed in the three countries where the epidemic was most concentrated (Fairhead 2016; Lee-Kwan et al. 2014; Rabelo et al. 2016). Although the effects observed in these countries are important, investigating whether such negative consequences were observed in the United States is essential for understanding the implications of the globalization of stigma for immigrant communities abroad. Among African immigrants in Dallas, the contexts in which these effects were observed varied. They included social interactions between individuals and interactions between the public and African immigrant institutions. Compared to what we know of the effects of stigma on the welfare of individuals, very little is known about its effects on immigrant institutions. As such, it is important to understand the ways in which the stigma of Ebola affected immigrant businesses, churches, and other social institutions in the African immigrant community.

Therefore, to build a complete portrait of African immigrants' experiences with stigma, a number of questions need to be answered, such as: What strategies were used to promote the narrative of blame used to target these immigrants with stigma? How were their experiences with the stigma of Ebola related to the tendency of linking epidemics to local and global places? To what extent did these experiences negatively affect life in their communities? Finally, did the stigma of Ebola affect national attitudes toward issues of immigration in general and that toward African immigrants in particular?

The Media, Ebola Fears, and the Otherization of Africans

Private fears about the spread of disease are usually associated with media reports on epidemics (Ridout et al. 2008; Scheufele 1999). However, the role of the media in influencing public fear of disease is much more extensive. Part of this involves its role in providing a critical mechanism for developing a common set of beliefs on the threat of disease. One way this is done is by promoting images of notable cases of infection, which are inadvertently used to construct stereotypes that target specific groups at risk. After the Ebola outbreak in Dallas, these dynamics became fully functional in subsequent news reports. As part of this process, the role of the media was extended to the implicit identification of subjects who could be viewed as potential sources of risk. Playing into the hands of public ignorance about Africa and its cultures, the media produced an image of Africa that was informed by stereotypes of its backwardness, poverty, and disease. Unknowingly, therefore, it constructed an image of African identity that was similar to that developed in imperial Britain during its quest to civilize the so-called primitive peoples of the south (Bonsu 2009; Cohen 2015). The specific strategies used to develop the distorted image of Africa varied. They included the routine integration of Africa into media reports that unwittingly disseminated a fear of the virus as well as the misrepresentation of African cultural symbols in ways that promoted an image of backwardness.

Monson (2017) suggests that the use of these strategies became more frequent after Duncan's diagnosis was confirmed. Her analysis of the language of news headlines during this period reveals a clear shift from neutral reporting of the epidemic to the transmission of emotional messages linked with fear (Monson 2017).* Across the globe, international media reports provided the main means for advancing a related global narrative of fear and, together with the domestic media, provided the main framework through which the risk of Ebola was understood (Cohen 2015). The virus was thus presented as being from Africa at the same time that it was

---

* This increase in fear was also implied in trends in Google searches. While searches for the word "Ebola" were relatively insignificant in March 2014, they peaked around the second week in October, following the death of Thomas Duncan (Cohen 2015).

being described as lethal (Monson 2017). Moreover, Ebola was so lethal that its risks were not only compared to those posed by biological weapons but to the worst of these weapons (Cole 2014). A CNN report, for example, referred to the virus as the ISIS of biological agents (Al-Jabban 2014). However, this narrative discounted the voices of experts who frequently argued that the risk of contracting Ebola was much lower than what was perceived (Kim et al. 2016). As these risks were promoted, the perceived connection between Africa and Ebola took on a life of its own. Public reactions to these reports thus became similar to the hysteria observed during the 1995 Ebola outbreak in Zaire (Ungar 1998).

Along with the incorporation of Africa into the dissemination of fear, the interpretation of media reports was conducted through a prism characterized by a misrepresentation of African cultures and its peoples. This was seen in the devaluation of African cultural symbols, the promotion of misinformation about its cultural practices, and the ascription of other undesirable traits to African people. A key part of this process involved linking the Ebola epidemic with Africans' distrust of Western medicine and their supposedly mysterious cultural practices (Cohen 2015; Monson 2017). For example, one Fox News commentator claimed that Africans in Ebola-affected countries could arrive in the United States on a plane after seeking treatment from a witch doctor who practiced Santeria* (Farhi 2014; Rothkopf 2014). Another cultural misrepresentation was found in a news article published by the *Daily Beast*, which attempted to highlight the apparent backwardness of African culture under the headline "Kissing the Corpses in Ebola Country" (Haglage 2014). The kissing practice it describes was one found in Uganda, East Africa, which is not only more than five thousand miles away from the source of the West African Epidemic but was also Ebola-free at that time. A final example was the racist representation of Africans seen in a front-page picture of a chimpanzee by *Newsweek* along with a headline implying that Africans could bring Ebola to the United States by smuggling bush meat into the country (Flynn and Scutti 2014). To be sure, many of these attempts to racialize African culture were criticized by other commentators (McGovern 2014; Monson

* One of the problems with this claim is that Santeria is widely practiced in the Caribbean and not necessarily in Africa.

2017); however, they were important for confirming the worst stereotypes about Africans held by Americans.

Against the backdrop of these stereotypes, a wide range of African cultural markers, including food, apparel, and languages, were used as tools for identifying the targets of stigma. In light of the hysteria created by the media, public fears about being infected resulted in the identification of a broad range of possible suspects who could be stigmatized. This targeting process could not just be limited to Duncan—because Ebola was a disease that was believed to be "all over Africa" (Monson 2017), anyone from the continent who looked like him was considered a potential threat. After all, they had a geographic connection to the continent, had similar racial characteristics as Duncan, and were presumed to be associated with the same set of primitive cultural practices that promoted the spread of disease.

It was these caricatures of Africa, provided by the media, that underscored the media's role in the otherization of Africans during the epidemic. Otherization in this sense refers to the construction of an image of Africans as racialized others in the process that distinguished them from mainstream America. It involves the creation of social demarcations between out-groups and in-groups in a way that identifies the former as an alien "other" used to make a distinction between "them" and "us" (Monson 2017). "Them" in this case refers to Africans in the sense that they were un-American, and because they were not "us," it was easy to blame them for the spread of a foreign disease. As noted in one prior study, the otherization of out-groups during epidemics helps to provide a false sense of immunity to in-groups by projecting the threat of infection to the racialized "other" (Cohen 2015). In part, this was seen in reports that framed the Ebola outbreak as being "in that part of the world" while at the same time describing it as being "out of control" (Paradzai 2015). For the otherization of Africans to be complete, it also needed to have geographic dimension. Thus, as a result of flawed notions of Africa that were held by many members of the public, this dimension involved collapsing the boundaries between the three affected countries in West Africa and those of the other fifty-one Ebola-free countries on the continent to form a single entity. In the process, African immigrants from Liberia, Sierra Leone, and Guinea became indistinguishable from their counterparts from countries such as Rwanda, Mozambique, and Kenya.

A final factor that contributed to the emerging narrative on Africans was the attention given to sources of misinformation about Ebola itself. For example, analysis of Ebola-related rumors on Twitter following Duncan's death revealed that the most prevalent of these was one that reinforced the racialized narrative on the disease (Jin et al. 2014). It was the belief that the Ebola vaccine only worked on people who were White. People who depended on social media as a source of information were thus exposed to descriptions of Africans that presented them as being different. These messages underscored the notion of the inferiority of African heritage while reinforcing the distinction between Black Africans and the American mainstream. It was no different than those messages found in societies that use cultural stereotypes to promote distorted perceptions about the health of ethnic minorities. Furthermore, in the United States it reflected the historical tendency to create social demarcation between people of African heritage and the rest of the public, and to advance public perception of their inferior health (Postell 1951).

All told, the narrative created by the media used various strategies to develop an ideological basis for stigmatizing African immigrants. It linked fear-filled reports of Ebola with perceptions of African countries as being undifferentiated. It promoted a presumed relationship between the threat of Ebola and African cultural symbols. Finally, it represented Africans as the racialized other who were different from mainstream Americans. When combined with reports that described the ease with which the virus is transmitted, this narrative provided a point of departure from which many people took action to address their fear of the disease.

Ebola Stigma and Social Lives of Africans in Dallas

At the outset of the outbreak, many Liberian immigrants were not immediately exposed to the brunt of these actions. However, their encounters with stigma became more frequent as the visual evidence of their connection with the outbreak increased. This became most notable after Liberian immigrant leaders shifted their strategy for addressing the media. When the outbreak started, it was easy for them to give separate interviews to individual journalists, but as interview requests increased, it made more sense for them to conduct news conferences, where they addressed multiple reporters in the same place. Nevertheless, there was a notable downside to these conferences. After George participated in one seen on national television, he became linked with the epidemic in ways that had negative consequences for his relationship with his coworkers. When he returned to work the next day, his normal routine was interrupted by his manager, who immediately summoned him to his office. After he arrived, George was asked a series of questions. What was his relationship with Duncan? Did he have any interaction with him before he became sick? George's manager was not just asking these questions because he was curious. Other employees had seen George on TV and expressed fears of being around him. While he was bothered by the questions, George still attempted to calm these fears with his responses. He observed that just as no one expects American leaders to have a personal relationship with each US citizen, it is wrong to assume that leaders in the Liberian community personally knew Duncan. He further explained that although he respected the concerns of his coworkers, he had a more important reason to avoid exposing himself to infected people—his family. George's response helped to allay the fears of his manager; however, the incident was instructive because it marked the first time he was stigmatized based on his perceived association with the city's first Ebola patient.

The stigma of Ebola was not experienced by George alone. In describing how they felt during the anti-African backlash following Duncan's death, many African immigrants framed their experiences in terms consistent with the notion that they were treated as untouchables. They described feeling like they were "looked down upon as if [they] were filthy," how they were treated as if they "came to America to spread diseases," and how locals "still looked at [them] like [they were] Ebola carriers or something." These accounts were based on subjective perceptions; however, they were backed by reports of specific interactions that were unquestionably associated with the process of being stigmatized. These included encounters with questions such as "Where are you from?" directed toward those perceived to be African, with a response such as "Liberia" or "Sierra Leone" being followed by reactions as explicit as "Oh my gosh, have you washed your hands?"

Even when reactions were more subtle, they still left little to the imagination concerning what the person asking the question was thinking. Take, for example, what happened when Beke, who was from Nigeria, and her friend from Sierra Leone visited a fast-food restaurant's drive-through. They were about to place their order at the window when the cashier recognized cultural clues that suggested that they were from Africa (i.e., they were talking to each other in a foreign language, and while placing their order they spoke to the cashier with a foreign accent). Using these markers, the cashier immediately stigmatized the two as potential Ebola carriers, as Beke describes in the following account:

> One of my friends, and he's actually from Sierra Leone, we went to the drive-through at McDonald's, and we ordered some food, and the cashier was like, "Hey. . ." You know, we were talking, you know how our English is? Well, it's broken English.* Right here in Dallas. Yeah. McDonald's right there on Cartwright, so we started talking in our broken English, and the guy already had the money from us. He was driving, my friend was driving, and [the cashier] asked the question, "Where are you guys from?" and [my friend] said, "I'm from Sierra Leone." Guess what [the cashier] did? He just dropped the money down, put on a pair of gloves, and picked the money up again. I was speechless. I didn't know what to say. I was SPEECHLESS. He dropped the money down. Oh, yeah, he dropped the money down, put on a pair of gloves, and he said, "I'm sorry, excuse me," and then he picked the money back up. I was like, "Did you see that?" "Excuse me. . ." So yeah, yeah, so it was crazy.

Such reactions from the public, according to another community resident, had just one explanation: "They are listening to the news." His own experience during this period taught him that speaking English with an accent in public attracted an immediate reaction from people who wanted to know where he was from. As he observed, however, Africans still attracted stigmatized reactions from the public, even in the absence of these vocal clues. This was because people were creating an image of risk associated with those who looked African and were acting out their fears accordingly. He explained that even when "you're in line in a grocery store, people choose not to come near you; they give you a little space and try to keep away from you" despite the fact that "they don't know who you are."

These encounters with stigma occurred in a range of social contexts.

---

* The language Beke is referring to is a form of pidgin English commonly spoken in West African countries such as Nigeria, Sierra Leone, Ghana, and Liberia.

For instance, George's experience with his manager was part of a large set of encounters with stigma faced by Africans at their places of employment. Around the community, there were accounts of people returning from visits to African countries such as Kenya who were asked by their employers to stay home from work. While such a response reflected the use of a reductionist view of Africa to identify potential targets of stigma, it was also associated with a stereotypical view of Africa as a place of disease, which was deceptively easy to deploy.

Other accounts of experiences with stigma at work were more direct and negatively affected the relationships between Africans and their coworkers. Sam faced such experiences while working at a job he combined with his work as a pastor of a small Liberian immigrant church. His coworkers, who knew he was from Liberia, did very little to hide their concerns about being around him. According to him, "they were scared to death." One of them, who usually tries to avoid anyone with minor ailments such as headaches, was particularly disturbed and specifically told Sam he did not want to be around him. Much later, it became clear that his coworkers' reactions were not so much driven by Sam's association with Liberia as a country but by perceptions of him as someone who regularly interacts with others in the Liberian community. In other words, his colleagues' fear of him was driven by his perceived association with the local outbreak, which made him a possible risk to those who feared Ebola.

Owing to the reductionist view of Africa held by many local residents, related encounters with stigma associated with the reactions of coworkers were also experienced by Africans from other countries. Two of the most unexpected of these involved Dr. Adu, an immigrant from Ghana. They were unexpected because they occurred at his office at a healthcare facility located not too far from Dallas. Dr. Adu was not only an accomplished professional with graduate degrees in different professional fields but was also the leading cardiologist* among the group of doctors at the facility.

The first encounter occurred a few weeks before Duncan arrived in Texas. At the time, the epidemic had already started in Guinea, Liberia, and

---

* His specific area of specialization is very rare and has been changed to protect his identity.

Sierra Leone. After receiving word that his elderly mother was seriously sick in Ghana, Dr. Adu immediately went home to see her. After he returned to Texas, however, he was surprised to notice signs of unease among his coworkers and patients. They were concerned that he may have been infected with Ebola, even though no case of the disease had been reported in Ghana during the epidemic. These fears were much higher among his patients than his colleagues. Consequently, they started calling to cancel their appointments to see him. However, he was not that bothered by the cancellations, because, as he maintained, it seemed like his patients "wanted to wait to see what was going to happen with me before deciding whether to see me or not."

The negative reaction toward Dr. Adu became more institutionalized in a second encounter, which occurred three months later, after his mother died. Once again, he traveled to Ghana, even though the Ebola epidemic was elsewhere in West Africa. After returning to the United States, he witnessed a response from his employer that was not only based in fear but, in Dr. Adu's view, had a limited basis in the practice of medicine. A senior colleague sent a memo to all doctors in the network describing what they were expected to do if they traveled to Africa. Any doctor returning from the continent, it explained, needed to be certified by a primary-care physician to show that they were Ebola-free before they would be allowed back to work. While the innuendo was clear, Dr. Adu was stunned. He was shocked to learn that the memo was sent by someone who was a doctor, because in his view "it [did] not show any level of science or [an understanding of] physiology." To emphasize his point, he explained that "there's just no way that a primary-care physician can certify that someone is Ebola-free." However, he continued, in order to confirm this notion, he did the following: "I got a copy of [the memo] and I sent it to our infectious disease specialist in town, one of the doctors here, to get his input and assessment of the protocol. He just laughed and laughed and said, 'This doesn't look very intelligent. If you have come up with some guidelines or a proposal for your people, you should at least either contact the CDC or somebody who has some knowledge about how to control diseases in the population or in a place and not just be based on paranoia.' So we just laughed at it."

Several things were clear from these experiences. First, an institutional response was generated to address the travels of professionals, like Dr. Adu, who had any connection with Africa and thus represented a risk of transmitting Ebola. Second, the concern of Ebola was so significant that an institutional response was triggered in ways that appeared to deviate from the professional standards used for determining whether someone was Ebola-free. As Dr. Adu further explained, the response possibly resulted from the need to do something to calm the fears of colleagues. They knew he was African and that he went to Africa during an epidemic. These two facts were enough to arouse their concerns, even though they were professionals in the field of healthcare.

Apart from these experiences, there were extensive reports of encounters with stigma among Africans at educational institutions. Some of the most explicit occurred within the Dallas Independent School District, where African immigrant children were viewed as carriers of Ebola. In these contexts, the stigma of the virus was deployed in various ways. It was seen, for example, in the decision of school officials who specifically asked African children to stay home from school out of concern that they could infect others with the virus. Around Vickery Meadow, parents with children who had African classmates were further concerned that the latter could have interacted with Duncan (Herskovitz 2014). In fact, some of them took action on their own rather than wait for an institutional response from the school district. After the superintendent of the district announced that five children were among a group of people believed to have had contact with Duncan, many parents in the community decided to keep their children away from school (Hanna 2014).

While these actions were somewhat understandable, they were compounded by additional measures taken by school officials who wanted to take action to allay the fears of parents. One example of this was an incident involving an African child whose family lived in the same apartment complex as Troh. Motivated by his desire to keep perfect attendance in school, the child continued to attend classes even after Duncan was diagnosed. Subsequently, however, he was asked to stay home by officials after his presence in school generated backlash among parents. What occurred next was an overreaction, a public relations exercise that only served to reinforce the image of African children as being infected with disease.

Lydia, who worked with children in the community at the time, recalled how the exercise unfolded:

The Dallas Independent School District came in with hazmat teams to clean the schools. And they knew it wasn't necessary, they did it to appease the families, but they made a big show of it and had it on television and everything else: "The hazmat teams are in the school." Well, yeah, okay, that may have made parents feel better, but it also made people feel like, "Oh, that's the school with the hazmats; it's so bad there, they had to have the hazmat team." There was just so much misunderstanding of the disease and how it's spread and everything.

As important as these institutional responses were in creating an image of African children as being contaminated, they did comparatively less harm than the backlash they received from their peers. As she continued to provide details of other encounters with stigma faced by African children, Lydia discussed two incidents that involved student athletes from a local high school. In one, players from a visiting high school team refused to shake hands with these students, who included Africans, because they were afraid of contracting Ebola. In the second incident, the local players went to a fast-food restaurant after the game but were reportedly refused service. And it did not end there. Encounters with stigma were also reported among children in African families outside Dallas. One such encounter was a case of stigma-related bullying at a school in the Bronx. In that community, two brothers from Senegal, Amadou and Pape Drame, were taunted with shouts of "Ebola" by schoolmates who beat them up on the school's playground (Hagan 2014).

African students at postsecondary institutions were not excluded from these stigmas, although their experiences were less extreme. At Navarro College, about sixty miles from Dallas, two Nigerian students were refused admission on the grounds that Ebola cases had been recorded in their country (Jones 2014). Furthermore, there were stigmas encountered by African students in their classrooms. In the case of Saran, an immigrant from Ivory Coast, it occurred while taking a class required for her certification as a healthcare worker. Her classmates, who understood that there were differences among African countries, used her country of origin to treat her quite differently from a South African student who was also in her class. It started with classmates asking her how far Ivory Coast was from Liberia. When she responded that the countries share a border, she observed a notable decline in the way her classmates interacted with her compared to their interaction with her South African classmate.

Other experiences with stigma, however, were not as restricted to specific institutional contexts. Arguably the most compelling of these was that of Louise Troh and her family. In an effort to contain the local spread of Ebola, health officials had placed them in quarantine after Duncan was diagnosed with the disease. After subsequent tests confirmed that they had no trace of the virus, they were allowed to return to their normal lives. However, life for the Troh family was anything but normal. Their belongings were destroyed by the hazmat teams that decontaminated their apartment, and to top things off, their old apartment complex did not want them to return at the end of the quarantine (Troh 2015). Their search for another apartment to rent was made difficult by their association with Duncan. Indeed, this association was the ultimate stigmatizing attribute, and for this reason, despite the fact that they were medically cleared of the virus, no one wanted to rent them an apartment.

Leading the task of helping them find a new home was Susan, who worked at a church the family attended. She reported witnessing the systematic stigmatization of the family by renters who refused to allow them on their premises.* Each apartment complex they contacted declined their application, with some of them being very explicit about why the family was unwanted. According to Susan, every area basically said, "You can apply here, but you need to know that we're not going to accept [your] application." Although this admission was not made directly to Troh, she still recognized why her rental applications were being rejected. At one point, she frustratingly conceded that "I have this Ebola stigma on me and no one will take me in" (Blake and Robinson 2014). In the end, her church replaced many of the possessions they lost when their apartment was decontaminated and found an organization that provided housing for the family. However, even these efforts were criticized by those who argued

---

* The apartment complexes that rejected the family were mainly located around the Vickery Meadow neighborhood. After being released from quarantine, Duncan's fiancée wanted her family to return to the neighborhood because they were familiar with it and it was the neighborhood where her kids went to school (Troh 2015).

that the family could not have lost that much in the first place because they were refugees (Troh 2015).

As disconcerting as these encounters with stigma were, they were viewed by African immigrants from a wide range of perspectives. At one end were reactions of shock and anger at the demeaning ways in which Africans were treated, including Beke's disappointment with the way she was treated at the drive-through. Conversely, there was a surprising degree of rationalization of the generalized fear of Africans by those who had themselves been the victims of stigma. It was not clear whether these reactions were used as a way of coping with the consequences of stigma. However, they included arguments that explained these experiences as a reflection of American ignorance and a general lack of knowledge about Africa. For example, Kiragu, whose relief donations were rejected by refugees at Vickery Meadow, argued that these reactions were understandable. Given that the public knew the disease originated in Africa, he reasoned, it was not surprising that locals assumed that there was more than a 50 percent chance that an African had the disease rather than someone who looked Asian. Another argument was that the stigma of Ebola was driven by paranoia. For Josiah, a Sierra Leonean who had similar experiences, the American public became

> paranoid because of the way the Ebola virus was described, and the way it was labeled to be killing people, its viciousness; it made people paranoid, of course, and you don't blame these people. Some of them are not as diverse as you and I are. You know? That's why I was not so worried because we've seen so [much] other stuff in the past, so many other bad things. Yeah, should they be trying to say all Africans are bad or Africans should be set aside in a separate area? No, I don't think that's a good thing, but you have to understand where these people are coming from as well.

Placism, Racism, and the Stigma of Ebola

There is no question that those who deployed the stigma against Africans in Dallas had a simplistic, inaccurate view of Africa. In some cases, the threat posed by Africans was perceived to be connected with residents who lived around the community of Vickery Meadow. These observations raise important questions about the extent to which the stigma of Ebola was connected to specific geographic places. What, for example, was the relative significance of perceptions of Africa and of Vickery Meadow in the deployment of stigma? Were residents of the neighborhoods of Nina Pham and Amber Vinson stigmatized to the same extent as residents of Vickery Meadow? How were place-specific stigmas combined with a racialized view of Africa to construct the threat posed by Africans beyond the borders of Texas?

Such questions are usually addressed by analysts examining the significance of placism. The term "placism" was developed to understand the discrimination and marginalization experienced by disadvantaged groups such as ethnic minorities who live in poor communities. Placism, which is also referred to as prejudice of place (Palmer 2011), thus features prominently in accounts of how stigmas are developed and deployed based on where people live (Evans 2016; Jimerson 2005; Sernhede 2014).

After the outbreak in Dallas, therefore, it provided a critical perspective from which disparities in the deployment of stigmas were examined. One study by Smith-Morris (2017) examines these differences by exploiting the contrast between the neighborhood characteristics of Duncan and Nina Pham to assess whether there were variations in the general response to the virus. Compared to Duncan, who lived in Vickery Meadow, Pham lived in an affluent, predominantly White neighborhood located on M Street. Notably, Smith-Morris (2017) found that while residents of Pham's neighborhood reported that they did not feel stigmatized by Ebola, their predominantly Black African counterparts in Vickery Meadow reported that they did. Based on these findings, she concluded that the stigma experienced by residents of Vickery Meadow was not explained by the fact that their neighborhood itself was more stigmatized compared to that of M Street. The differences, she argued, were more of a reflection of the stigmatization of Africa as a racialized place rather than of neighborhood-related stigma. This conclusion is partly inconsistent with what one would expect given the existence of stereotypes of Vickery Meadow in the city. However, it underscores the importance of race for assessing differences in how the stigma of Ebola was deployed across neighborhood contexts.

Few people would disagree that the lack of encounters with stigma among the predominantly White residents of M Street may have been related to their relative position in the US racial hierarchy. Perspectives on racial inequality were thus routinely used by community residents to explain differences in the reaction toward Duncan and Nina Pham. According to one resident, people in the "mostly White, upscale" M Street area were treated differently in ways that continued to be evident several months after the death of Duncan. While locals "still relate Ebola to Vickery Meadow," she observed, they do not relate it to "M Street, where [Pham] lived, [which] also was like the [Village Apartments], where the other nurse lived." To a critical observer, however, these differences raise an important question: if the stigma of Ebola was exclusively driven by fear of the virus, why were similar patterns of stigmatized behavior not observed in the neighborhoods of each of the infected persons in the city?

In part, the answer lies in the fact that African immigrants' experiences with stigma reflected a combination of both a disadvantage tied to their racial minority status *and* a specific strand of placism known as epidemiological placism (Smith-Morris 2017). The latter refers to disease-related prejudices tied to a specific place, which in this case Smith-Morris suggests is Africa. These two factors explained why it was Black African bodies that were racialized as being infected with disease and not those of White residents in other neighborhoods.

Because this racialized version of epidemiological placism was not necessarily tied to Dallas, the stigmatization of African immigrants soon extended beyond the borders of the city. When it did, the stigma of Ebola broke loose from its initial association with residents of Vickery Meadow, where Duncan lived, to become more associated with the people connected to the place where he was from. There is an abundance of evidence showing the role of the latter in facilitating acts of discrimination against Africans elsewhere during the epidemic. In New Jersey, two children from Rwanda scheduled to start elementary school were asked to stay home by school officials (Chang 2014). In making this decision, school officials failed to recognize that there was no Ebola outbreak in Rwanda or that Rwanda is located farther from Guinea, Liberia, and Sierra Leone than New York is from California. In Pennsylvania, a young soccer player from Guinea was bullied with chants of "Ebola" by fans of the opposing team despite the fact that he had been in the United States for more than three years (Molinet 2014). There was also a case in Minnesota where a more general racialized view of African origins was used to ostensibly identify a

potentially infected person. It involved a call received by the state's department of health from a woman who reported that there was a Black man
wearing rubber gloves at a supermarket, after which she asked officials to
come "get him" (Almendrala 2015). Without knowing whether he was from
Africa, she simply used his racial characteristics to identify him as someone potentially infected with the disease.

Outside the United States, some of the most notable acts of Ebola-
related discrimination against Africans were observed in Europe. German
soccer fans were reported to have chanted "Ebola, Ebola" as an opposing
Black soccer player from Ghana was about to enter the field (Obermueller and Waters 2014). There were also at least two reported cases of such
stigma-related incidents in Italy. The first involved a three-year-old girl
from Uganda, who was asked to stay home from school because authorities feared that she had the disease, while the second was the experience
of a Guinean immigrant who was beaten by fellow passengers as she got
off a bus. The passengers claimed that she had Ebola (Laccino 2014). However, none of these incidents matched the racist attitudes expressed about
Africans by far-right French politician Jean-Marie Le Pen. A firm critic of
immigration, she lauded the possibility that Ebola deaths in Africa could
actually have a positive influence because it would help control what she
believed to be the surge in African immigration to France (Obermueller
and Waters 2014).

Ebola Stigma and Its Influence on African Immigrant Institutions

Taken together, these examples demonstrate the negative implications
that the stigma of Ebola had for the social lives of individuals. Another
perspective on these implications is represented by the increasing recognition of the effects of these stigmas on social institutions (Sartorius 2007).
These implications reflect the effects of stigma on members of these institutions as well as on that of more general stigmas that undermine the
ability of institutions to perform their functions. What we know about the
effects of these stigmas is, however, limited to analyses that focus on a
small set of issues, such as the strategies used by institutions to counter
health-related stigmas (e.g., Chin et al. 2008). A few attempts have also

been made to understand how ethnic institutions such as immigrant-owned restaurants are stigmatized during epidemics (Eichelberger 2007). However, rarely do they provide extensive accounts of how the customs, roles, and functions of institutions are affected by the stigma of disease.

In the weeks following the Ebola outbreak in Dallas, the diversity of ethnic institutions in the African community provided a rich set of targets for the public to stigmatize. Identifying these targets was relatively easy because of their association with cultural symbols of Africanness. These were symbols associated with the provision of cultural products (e.g., African food), the social characteristics of their workers, and the ethnic profiles of their clients. African-owned businesses were among the institutions most negatively affected by the stigma of Ebola, and there were several reasons for this. Many of them, including restaurants, hair salons, and grocery markets, provided services that involved physical contact with their clients. In addition, these businesses were small-scale enterprises with limited resources, which means that they were highly vulnerable to fluctuations in demand for their services. Owing to the visible presence of African workers at these institutions, it was also easy to employ the same stereotypes used to stigmatize African individuals to stigmatize these businesses as places to avoid.

Few businesses were as exposed to these vulnerabilities as African hair-braiding salons. The services they provide are culturally specific and require hours of physical contact with the bodies of their clients. The simplest hairstyles, for example, require one hair-braider to touch the head of her client, while cases that are more complex require two or more hair-braiders touching a client's head at the same time. Therefore, when the Ebola outbreak occurred in the city, Onike, who worked at a salon close to Vickery Meadow, immediately knew that it would be bad for business. As she put it, "I knew one way or the other, it was going to affect us here too." Her plight was complicated by her tendency to receive appointments over the phone; because she spoke with a heavy African accent, her conversations with her clients left little doubt about her association with the African cultural markers of risk.

It did not take long for Onike's suspicions to be confirmed. Clients who called the salon asked specific questions about what part of Africa she was from, and some of them canceled their appointments after learning that she was from Nigeria, in West Africa. She summed up the disturbing experience in the following account:

> I had at least six people that called me over the phone. They wanted to make an appointment to come do their hair. I guess they were new clients. The first thing they asked me was, "Are you from Africa?" I said, "Yes." "What part of Africa?" I said, "West Africa." "Okay, I will call you back," and they never called back. And then, some people when they're coming here, they ask me, "When was the last time you went home?" I mean, I just told them that I hadn't been home for the past year. Some of them will sit down and do their hair; some will still say, "I will come back." I had two clients who left.

Similar experiences were reported by other immigrant hair-braiders from West Africa. One of these was Binta, an immigrant from Guinea who owned a small shop on the other side of town, where she operated a hair-braiding salon and sold African fabrics. Not only did she have clients who canceled their appointments, but she also saw a decline in sales as fewer customers stopped by to patronize her business. The decline in support was sometimes dramatic. One estimate from California indicated that patronage of African hair-braiding salons declined from about five customers per day to one per week due to fears of contracting Ebola (Baba 2014).

Like hair-braiders, transport operators directly interact with their clients, although their degree of physical contact with them is more limited. These interactions, however, made airport shuttle operators more vulnerable to the negative consequences of stigma. Alim, who was from Liberia, explained that part of this was due to clients' response to their accents, which identified them as Africans. While discussing the discrimination they faced during the crisis, he used himself as an example to highlight the economic effects of stigma. In order to conceal his identity, he tried to talk as little as possible after picking up clients at the DFW airport. Occasionally, however, this strategy was compromised by customers who specifically wanted to know where he was from. Responding that he was Liberian led many customers to stop using his services. These actions not only hurt his feelings but also his wallet.

According to informants in the community, the stigma of Ebola did not have much of a negative effect on the operations of African grocery stores.

Perhaps this was because they are small establishments mainly patronized by other Africans in the city. In other states, the effects of the outbreak on African grocery businesses were quite significant. The most notable was observed in the open market in an area known as Little Liberia in Staten Island, New York. Most of the market vendors were from Liberia, and they sold African products such as palm oil, dried fish, spices, and locally grown vegetables. Three weeks after the death of Duncan, the number of vendors in the market declined, from about twenty-two in the previous months to five (CBS 2014). The decrease was partly due to the difficulty of getting access to suppliers, but it also resulted from a decline in patronage from customers. Some of these customers lived in the community and may have observed African residents being subjected to frequent harassment by locals, who yelled at them to "go back to Africa with your Ebola" (CBS 2014; Shen 2014).

Other social institutions in the African immigrant community were less affected by the stigma of Ebola than African-owned businesses. Some of these effects were observed in churches, several of which experienced a decline in attendance. Not surprisingly, the most dramatic effects were observed in social institutions whose activities revolved around physical contact among people. These institutions included soccer teams, which provide a major source of recreation for African males in the Dallas area. One of these teams included players from Liberia and Sierra Leone. When Sama, a team leader from Sierra Leone, discussed how the team had been affected, it was difficult to miss the undertones of fear in his account. He started by indicating that all team practices were suspended during the outbreak, which negatively affected the team's training for local competitions. However, as he further explained, the decision was motivated by a fear of contracting the virus from a specific group of players. As he put it, "We were scared because the Liberians always mingled with us because we were buddy buddies." When the situation improved, however, the team resumed its normal activities but with new precautions to limit the possibility of transmitting the virus from one sweaty teammate to another.

Ebola Fears and the Complicated Nature of Stigma

Sama's response is important because it suggests that limiting our understanding of the stigma of Ebola to acts of discrimination committed by others against Africans provides an incomplete picture of the dynamics of stigma during the outbreak. As already discussed, there is no doubt that the backlash against African immigrants may have been associated with their status as racial minorities. At the same time, in the context of extreme fear of Ebola, more complex trajectories of stigmatization were observed. They involved the deployment of stigma by individuals who belonged to the same groups that local natives targeted for stigma. This suggests that, even among minority groups blamed for the spread of disease, stigmas can be deployed through processes that identify potential threats of infection using other markers of risk.

The most common marker used to form these alternative trajectories was Liberian nationality. Unlike many members of the public who saw Africans as an undifferentiated population, African immigrants generally could differentiate between members of the various national groups in their community. On the one hand, the use of Liberian nationality as a marker of risk was surprising because Liberia was not the only West African country affected by the epidemic. On the other hand, however, it was intuitive. First, immigrants from Liberia were seen as a more immediate threat because they were perceived as having had the most contact with Duncan before his diagnosis compared to other Dallas residents. Second, they were targeted by a narrative of blame that held them responsible for the general backlash against Africans in the city. One of them captured this pattern of blame when he described the response he received from his African coworkers as follows: "You go to work [and] they tell you, 'It's because of you that now all Africans have been classified as a problem, so don't come around me.'"

Besides Liberian nationality, stigma deployment within the African community further involved the use of other markers of risk. Among the most useful was relationship proximity with Duncan. Accordingly, even among Liberians, some of the highest levels of stigma targeted those perceived as having had a close relationship with him. The biggest threat of all was Louise Troh. She was blamed by other Liberians for her apparent role in the start of the outbreak, and they were deliberate in letting her know how they felt. She was asked questions such as "Isn't our life hard enough already? Why did you bring that man here? Why did that man come to America?" (Troh 2015, 153).

Troh's ordeal was only a small part of the layered patterns of stigma experienced within segments of the Liberian and Sierra Leonean communities. Sam, who was from Liberia, maintained that at one point Liberians were even afraid to associate with Liberian churches, and that Sierra Leoneans he knew were afraid of other Sierra Leoneans. According to him, the fear was pervasive because "they didn't know who was whom." They did not know whom to trust, who had just returned from countries affected by the epidemic, or how to differentiate between infected and noninfected persons. What was most disappointing for Sam was the way Liberians stigmatized Troh's apartment as an Ebola-infected place. He described the reason for this as follows: "The first case of Ebola coming to America was the Duncan story, so you can imagine. Everybody who knew that family automatically got to the corner [and said] 'Eh, don't go around that family. He was there in that house.' That house was like a . . . how do you call it? [They thought that] you were walking into an Ebola camp if you went to that house."

Other stigmas among Africans were driven by the fear of other African residents of Vickery Meadow. These fears suggest that neighborhood placism still played a role in the deployment of stigmas by Africans themselves. The stigma against these residents was mainly found among Africans with some kind of relationship with the community. One of them, a resident of the area, reported having had a fear of driving on streets close to Troh's apartment and frequently receiving calls from friends pleading with her to avoid the area near the apartment.

Similar fears were expressed by Africans who lived in the suburbs. Josiah, for example, lived away from Vickery Meadow but occasionally went there to visit relatives he had brought to the United States from Sierra Leone. After learning that Duncan lived in the neighborhood while he was infected, Josiah stopped visiting his relatives out of concern for his immediate family. Describing the steps he took to avoid the area, he made the following observations:

> What I did was—and I did that myself and for my children, of course—there was a specific location that the patient actually resided. At the time, Thomas Duncan—if you believe the name of the gentleman—he was a Liberian by nationality. He was residing in the Park Lane area,* which we call in Dallas the

---

* The Park Lane area is in the general area of Vickery Meadow. Some people use the two names interchangeably.

United Nations because you have so many nationalities residing in this particular area. . . . So I tried not to drive around that vicinity at all, and I told my children, I said: "Make sure you don't go in that [area]," because we have relatives staying in that area. A few years ago, we brought some relatives here to the States. Some of them live over there. We told them to be careful.

Each of the three markers used in the deployment of stigma among Africans—national origin, relationship proximity, and association with Vickery Meadow—was somewhat intuitive. At the same time, there were other instances of the deployment of stigma by Africans that were less so, and they underscored the unpredictable ways in which targets of stigma are identified when fear of infection is significant.

Joyce, an immigrant from Sierra Leone, for example, was still confused about why her family was stigmatized by a close friend who was from Liberia. Joyce was a highly trained public health professional who did not travel to Africa during the epidemic and knew what she needed to do to avoid contact with people who were possibly infected. She had cultivated a strong relationship with her friend from Liberia and was willing to take risks to maintain the relationship. One example of this was when her friend's daughter returned from Liberia at the start of the epidemic. Joyce allowed her friend's daughter to come over to her house after she expressed a desire to visit. Describing how her family responded at the time, she said: "We didn't say, 'Oh no, you've been to Liberia, [and] there is Ebola there. Don't come to our house and so and so.' We were just okay with it." A few weeks later, Joyce's friend saw her as a target, and this made Joyce very upset. Her friend's rationale was simple—Joyce's family attended social events with other Africans in the city, so being around her posed a potential threat of infection. The irony was not lost on Joyce as she described what occurred: "She started saying, 'Oh, I'm not coming to your house until this whole thing ends because you guys go to parties and things like that.' And can you imagine, we could have been dead. Her child came from there, and came straight to [my] house. We were still friendly; we didn't reject her or say, 'No, don't come to our house,' but that was their reaction. So I respected it. I guess we're not the reactive type of people, so we didn't react as much as they did."

Other Implications of the Stigmatization of Africans

Outside the community, public hostility toward Africans continued to have wider implications that extended beyond its influence on their lived experiences, on the operations of their institutions, and on social interactions among themselves. As shown in the recent history of epidemics associated with immigrants, these periods can trigger political responses that further stigmatize them in ways that are subsequently followed by backlash. Some of these responses involve political leaders capitalizing on sentiments of fear to push for policies that restrict immigration. Indeed, this notion of immigrants as a threat to public health was invoked to develop some of the earliest exclusionary policies, including the US Immigration Act of 1891. Congress passed the act in a social context defined by political concerns about the need to protect America from disease outbreaks in other countries (Chishti et al. 2014). Since then, this protection rationale has remained a central part of campaigns aiming to restrict immigration from specific regions of the world, including Asia, Africa, and the Caribbean.

Political rhetoric used to promote these campaigns exploits negative stereotypes held by the public to construct an image of immigrants as the racialized other. It includes calls for banning people with loathsome diseases and requirements for immigrants to undergo physical and mental health assessments (Markel and Stern 2002). Anti-immigration activists also use periods of epidemic to call on leaders to protect the American way of life from being polluted by immigration from poor countries (Markel and Stern 2002). Such stigma-laden rhetoric remained relevant among political leaders advocating for immigration control based on fears that immigrants are carriers of infectious diseases.

Anti-African sentiments during the Ebola crisis thus provided rich fodder to those who wished to control immigration from Africa and politicize the national debate on immigration. For example, a popular conservative talk show host linked the outbreak in Dallas with the issue of undocumented immigration by claiming that there were large numbers of undocumented immigrants in the affected Liberian immigrant community (Bernstein 2014). Other political leaders tapped into the latent fear of the disease in ways that exploited the wider emotional response to advocate for specific policies (Casey 2015). These actions were strategic and shaped by the timing of Duncan's death, which coincided with the midterm election campaigns (Hollibaugh 2017). Duncan's death was thus associated with a spike in Republican campaign adverts blaming the poor handling of the crisis on Democrats (Greer and Singer 2017).

While African immigrants received support from many political leaders during this period,* the stigma toward them was insinuated in the messages conveyed by politicians. Thom Tillis, a Republican representative who was running for the Senate in North Carolina, suggested that the outbreak in Africa could cause "bad actors" to come across the border while linking this to the need for more concrete action to seal and secure the border (Sargent 2014). Scott Brown, during his campaign to represent New Hampshire in the Senate, similarly called for travel restrictions against passengers from West Africa (Sargent 2014), even though experts consistently maintained that such restrictions would do little to stop the spread of the virus. Additionally, Bruce Braley, a Democratic representative from Iowa, called for all options to be put on the table to address the outbreak, including making changes in the admission of travelers at all American airports (Dunham 2014).

Polls indicating that measures such as travel bans were supported by the majority of Americans provided motivation for more calls for institutionalized action targeting Africans (Fuller 2014). Two weeks after the death of Duncan, Senator Marco Rubio (R-FL) expressed his intention to draft legislation that would immediately ban the Department of State from issuing visas to nationals of Guinea, Liberia, and Sierra Leone, as well as to those from countries where a significant number of Ebola cases had been diagnosed (Chishti et al. 2014). A similar measure was supported by Robert Goodlatte (R-VA), who was the chair of the House Judiciary Committee (Bennett 2014). In a rare show of bipartisan support for action, Democrats also developed their own proposals for addressing the issue of African immigration. Representative Alan Grayson (D-FL) made a request to the

---

* One of the best examples of this was seen in the actions of Dallas County Judge Clay Thompson. More details on this and of the positive role of public institutions are provided in chapter 7.

Secretaries of the Department of Homeland Security and the Department of State for similar bans (Nelson 2014), while Andrew Cuomo, the Democratic governor of New York, maintained that the government should seriously consider a ban (Berman 2014).

Faced with increased calls to restrict African immigration, the Obama administration took a number of steps that, ironically, made the president a target of the backlash. Rather than impose a travel ban, the administration argued against it on the grounds that it would hurt rather than help efforts to tackle the epidemic. What it did instead was to require all Africans traveling from affected countries to the United States to fly into one of five major airports, where enhanced screening measures were administered (Bennett 2014). Because the administration resisted calls to impose a travel ban, critics seized the opportunity to extend the racialization of the threat of Ebola in a way that otherized the president as being un-American (Abeysinghe 2016). This does not imply that the overall response of the administration was without fault. Its decision to send material support to help in the fight against the epidemic in Liberia was made a little later than expected. Moreover, it was arguably responsible for the inadequate preparation of the US healthcare system to treat Ebola cases such as that of Duncan.

Still, it is difficult to ignore how the threat of Ebola was racialized to target the president in order to serve broader political purposes. Accordingly, the president's actions were viewed as an attempt to show solidarity with people of his race. One commentator argued that "his affinity, his affiliations are with them, not us" (Abeysinghe 2016). Other critics used the opportunity to extend conspiracy theories that the president was not born in the United States and promoted a connection between him and Ebola on Twitter under the hashtag #Obola (Duhaime-Ross 2014). Coined by a conservative pundit, the term "Obola" had its origins in claims that the spread of Ebola to the United States was due to the administration's apparent open borders policy (Nolan and Cohen 2014). As support for this view increased on Twitter, critics extended the use of the #Obola hashtag to comments and images that linked the president with infectious diseases, primitive representations of Africans, and other racist caricatures.

Nevertheless, over time the stigma targeting African immigrants became central to attempts to reframe the national debate on undocumented immigration. Capitalizing on the public's reaction to the crisis, some critics offered the view that undocumented immigrants entering the United States are also likely to bring with them infectious diseases such as Ebola (Chishti et al. 2014). Stretching the argument further, one critic argued that even unaccompanied children traveling from Central and South America to the United States could threaten Americans by exposing them to the disease (Boerma 2014).

To put these reactions into perspective, it is important to observe that, as noted by Casey (2015), restrictive immigration policies are not always prejudicial; nevertheless, they can be exclusionary when they reinforce the otherization of groups considered to be outside the American mainstream. With regard to the political rhetoric observed during the Ebola outbreak, calls for such exclusions only helped to promote the perception of a divide between infected African bodies and clean bodies in America. In the process, they became part of the long history of the fear of contamination from Black bodies observed among the American public (Casey 2015).

Making Sense of African Immigrant Experiences

Life among African immigrants in Dallas was negatively affected by blame and stigma in the aftermath of the death of Duncan. Their social interactions were defined by experiences of discrimination, prejudice, and marginalization, while other reactions to their presence made it clear that they were seen as threats to public health. There is no doubt that these reactions were rooted in a generalized fear of Ebola. A focus on fear as the sole determinant of these experiences is nevertheless limiting because it understates the role of larger social forces in creating the conditions for linking the stigma of the virus to the characteristics of Black African bodies. This process was facilitated by the promotion of a narrative of difference based on an image of Africa as a place of epidemiological disaster. It was a narrative that invoked historical tropes of cultural dissimilarity based on a view of African immigrants as people with primitive traditions, such as their so-called reliance on witch doctors, which were so un-American that it put American communities at risk. By developing such a negative notion of Africanness, in a context where the origins of the Ebola epidemic were known to be in Africa, the stage was set for committing acts of discrimination against people who fit the profile of Africans. At the same time, this tendency of stigmatizing immigrants is not new and is consistent with what we know about the dynamics of stigma.

More generally, however, there were several notable features of the experiences of African immigrants during the outbreak in Dallas. First, they were labeled and targeted using diverse markers of risk. These included their speech patterns and their race. Moreover, those who used these markers to target Africans had a simplistic view of Africa that was generally inaccurate. These markers were also used in the racialization of the threat of Ebola in a way that extended the targeting of Africans beyond the United States. Along with racist stereotypes of Africa as a place of disease, the reductionist view of Africa as a single entity and its people as an undifferentiated population provided a basis for targeting even immigrants from countries unaffected by the virus for various acts of discrimination.

Second, there was no ambiguity among African immigrants that they were being stigmatized. They knew why this was happening and were aware of how they were being targeted. In some cases, such as in requests they received to wash their hands, the evidence of being stigmatized was too clear for them to miss.

Third, experiences of stigma had a negative effect on the social lives African immigrants. They resulted in a loss of status and in many cases were associated with a loss of resources. These negative experiences were also observed in their reduced opportunities for social interaction, but this is not surprising because such responses are frequently observed among people who are targets of stigma. Within the African immigrant community, systematic encounters with stigma did not just have implications for individuals but also for institutions. The institutions affected were mostly those that provided services requiring regular interaction with non-Africans. The negative consequences of stigma for these institutions were largely economic. Part of what made them important was that they illustrated the ways in which disease-related stigmas can undermine the operations of institutions central to the social and economic life of immigrant communities.

Finally, another feature of the stigma encountered by African immigrants was one that was somewhat different from those frequently observed in prior epidemics. It was the existence of multiple social pathways through which stigmas were deployed. These included vertical trajectories that involved local natives targeting African immigrants for acts of discrimination. However, they also included horizontal trajectories defined by experiences of stigma deployed by persons within the African immigrant community. In rare cases, it even included the deployment of stigma between persons of the same nationality. These experiences show that while the marginalization of out-groups by in-groups is important for stigmatization processes, out-groups can themselves employ processes of differentiation to create secondary patterns of stigma. For some groups, such as Liberian immigrants, therefore, the stigma of Ebola came from multiple sources. Their responses and those of other African immigrants are important for understanding whether they saw themselves as victims of the epidemic or whether these experiences were viewed as mere challenges to be overcome.

7 Fighting Back

Something unexpected happened in the midst of the backlash faced by Africans in the city. Parishioners from various churches began to meet to pray for an end to the outbreak. It was unexpected because of the circumstances under which it occurred. Church attendance had declined because of the fear of contracting Ebola. Moreover, the stigma of Ebola was still so intense that it discouraged many Africans from doing things that increased their interaction with the public. While their fears were real, these parishioners still came together to pray for a resolution to the crisis. It was a small way to begin the search for solutions, and this search focused on the outbreak in Dallas as well as the epidemic in West Africa. At the same time, the prayer meetings reflected the deep spirituality found in many African societies. When tragedies occur, people in these societies invariably turn to supernatural forces in their search for solace (Bangura 2016).

For many immigrants, therefore, this coordinated religious response was one of the most memorable actions they took in the aftermath of the outbreak. It was a response that was important for several reasons, one being that it served an instrumental purpose. It was structured around immigrants' faith in the ability of God to intervene on their behalf if they followed specific religious practices. When describing how these practices were employed, one parishioner referred to these periods as times when they prayed twice a day—from 9 a.m. to 10 a.m. and from 9 p.m. to 10 p.m.—and fasted. The prayers were offered for the safety of their relatives, for medical personnel taking care of the sick, and for those infected with the disease. Another instrumental purpose of this response was psychological. It helped those with relatives in West Africa to cope with their own fears. In fact, faith in God was cited as the driving force that kept them going during this period, and it was reflected in their frequent usage of phrases such as "we had God in us," "my strength was in God," or "God kept us."

Attending prayer meetings is also of theoretical significance because of its connection with the concept of bounded solidarity. In other words, it reflected the continued significance of collective shows of solidarity in the face of tragedy. Societies recovering from crises such as floods and tsunamis have long relied on this strategy as a means of promoting the cultivation of social capital needed for rebounding from tragedy (Plough et al. 2013; Sadeka et al. 2015). The task of recovering from the Ebola outbreak was similar. It required African immigrants to leverage the advantage of their common bonds and pay less attention to their social differences. As such, when Liberian churches organized prayer meetings, they focused on the collective needs of the community rather than on the goals of a specific church. The sense of community at these events was aptly captured by an attendee who acknowledged that they "did not care whose church [they] were going to, to do the prayers," and that they "did not care who was standing before [them]." They did this because, as he observed, "it was everybody's crisis." Under these circumstances, it was important to have a singular focus on the epidemic and the threat it posed. A similar sense of solidarity was found among Sierra Leonean immigrants, although they took it a step further by embracing their religious differences. While various Sierra Leonean immigrant churches held their own prayer meetings, members of their community also held interfaith events where Christian and Muslim leaders were invited to lead prayers. In so doing, they recognized the two dominant religions in the country and continued the long tradition of cooperation between the two religious groups, which is unlike that found in many countries in Africa.

More importantly, however, the prayer meetings were symbolic. They represented a determination to become more than just observers of the events that ripped through their city. Gathering together made them active participants who were willing to act to affect the outcome of these events. For these reasons, the prayer meetings also illustrated the agency of Africans in responding to the crisis. The meetings were a modest step that was part of a wider array of actions that demonstrated Africans' willingness to do what they could to change the course of the outbreak. Some of the first displays of such actions were observed before Duncan's arrival in the city, when Liberian and Sierra Leonean professionals met to lobby government officials in their home countries to stop the spread of the virus. Now that the threat of infection was more immediate and the negative consequences of stigma more apparent, there was a new sense of urgency to act to develop a more coherent set of responses.

These responses focused on three sets of issues. The first was on Ebola prevention and control, and it emerged as part of the effort to stop the local spread of the virus. It involved the development of proactive measures to promote positive health behaviors aimed at reducing the likelihood of more viral transmissions. The second focus was on the social consequences of the outbreak for African immigrants themselves. Addressing this objective involved taking steps to challenge the otherization of Africans and the narrative of blame that framed them as the human transmitters of the virus. The third focus was on their contributions to the global effort to control the epidemic in West Africa. It was based on the realization that although it was important to develop strategies to address the local crisis, it was also important to address the consequences of the epidemic faced by affected communities in Africa.

By addressing these issues, these immigrants showed why accounts of the social implications of epidemics that only focus on their negative consequences can be limiting. This is not to say that the negative consequences of these events should be ignored. Rather, it is to recognize that an acknowledgment of the proactive measures that were taken to address the challenges encountered during this period can help to provide a more well-rounded perspective on the responses observed during epidemics. This perspective is important because the ways in which communities respond to epidemics are much more diverse than is typically acknowledged. Communities affected by disease outbreaks not only react in fear to the possible threat of death but also develop ways to pick up the pieces and return to their normal lives. In order to reach this point, they take a series of counteractions to help them recover from their tragic experiences of fear. When these actions are discounted, however, we are forced to focus attention on their negative social experiences instead of developing a more comprehensive perspective on how they reacted.

Studies on immigrant experiences during epidemics that are affected by these issues have contributed to the emergence of an image that presents immigrants as powerless victims subjected to forces of xenophobia. In doing so, they understate the wealth of resources found in immigrant communities that can be used to help them recover from the consequences of tragedy. Among Africans in Dallas, for example, these resources were diverse. They included the social capital found in networks developed around their common identities as well as in the resources found in their ethnic institutions. Such patterns of collective identity and systems of social support are now recognized as fundamental determinants of the ability of communities to overcome periods of crisis (Plough et al. 2013). While ethnic institutions had traditionally provided similar resources to African immigrants, they were no doubt negatively affected by the disruption created by the outbreak. However, many of them continued to perform their core functions during this period and as a result were able to provide a foundation from which appropriate counteractions were taken. The main institutions involved in the process included the ethnic churches that organized the prayer meetings as well as cultural associations, humanitarian groups, and national-level organizations.

A less tangible asset found in the African immigrant community was their resilience. It was what allowed them to react to the obstacles they faced in the process of migrating to the United States. Before they arrived, it helped them deal with the horrors of civil conflict and economic hardship in Africa. After arriving in Dallas, it helped them to cope with the difficulty of separation from family members in their origin countries and to respond to the diverse shocks they experienced during their incorporation into society (Greeff and Holtzkamp 2007). Resilience also explained why the socioeconomic barriers they encountered after their arrival in Dallas did not always upend their efforts to live productive lives in the city.

As demonstrated earlier, African immigrants had further developed a wealth of experience in responding to adversity within their community. To be sure, none of these experiences were as challenging as the crisis they faced following the death of Duncan; however, these prior experiences were useful in other important ways. For example, their experiences with racism had helped them become familiar with what it means to be ostracized. The support they provided to those who were bereaved had helped them cultivate a tradition of helping individuals who faced personal tragedy. Moreover, their prior experiences with adversity had offered them opportunities for developing skills that were now useful in planning a response to the crisis. These skills had been developed in the systems of leadership found in their institutions, in planning fund-raising activities, and in creating the social infrastructure needed to support transnational humanitarian interventions in African societies.

How these skills were employed in their response to the consequences of the outbreak is a central part of the story of how marginalized communities recover from global health emergencies. However, these skills were not the only determinants of their ability to recover from the crisis. They were complemented by supportive actions taken by others outside their community in Dallas and by the actions of locals in Ebola-affected countries in Africa. Both sets of supportive actions were nevertheless taken at the behest of African immigrants, who took the responsibility of coordinating the overall response. A systematic accounting of the process is thus required to fully understand how this response ensued. What, for example, were the specific issues targeted by African immigrants in their response to the outbreak? How did they act to prevent the spread of Ebola in their community? To what extent did they draw on local natives in their attempt to mount a comprehensive response? Finally, how did they use transnational sources of social capital to address the process of recovery in Ebola-affected countries?

Evolving Responses to the Epidemic

At the outset of the outbreak, reactions to the spread of Ebola were mostly influenced by the belief that the crisis would be temporary. With few exceptions, therefore, the initial actions taken to respond to it were modest. Most of these actions sought to address its immediate implications for migrants themselves and for their families. The practical steps taken to meet these goals were simple: they ranged from the temporal suspension of plans to visit the affected countries to increasing communications with relatives in these contexts to encourage them to take the necessary precautions. While concerted action was limited, the slew of personal actions taken to deal with the crisis underscored the emergence of a resolve to refuse to allow the consequences of the epidemic to go unchecked.

Living through the backlash in Dallas increased the urgency to take additional action. It clarified the need to develop specific strategies for stopping the spread of the disease in Dallas despite the initial paralysis created by the fear of Ebola. Of critical importance was the need to promote the best practices used to control viral transmissions and to take appropriate action to enforce these practices. Next, action was needed to address the material consequences of the outbreak on the lives of community members such as Troh. It was not that the general stigma faced by other Africans was unimportant. In addition to the stigma faced by the Troh family, they were quarantined by authorities and had other pressing needs to address, which made them a priority, at least among Liberian immigrants. Then there was the international response to the crisis in West Africa. Unlike the local response, which targeted these diverse issues, the international response was generally less complex. Part of this was because the epidemic in West Africa started about a year prior to the Ebola outbreak in Dallas. As a result, enough evidence on the consequences of the epidemic abroad had been gathered, making it easy to develop a consensus around the need to help the communities it devastated in these contexts of poverty.

Ebola Prevention in the African Community

The earliest measures taken to address the local outbreak were those seeking to prevent the spread of Ebola within the African community. Following confirmation of Duncan's infection, the need to act increased with the uncertainty surrounding whether he had infected others in the city. No measures had been put into place to screen travelers arriving in the United States from Africa, and this gave rise to additional concerns that immigrants arriving from the continent represented an immediate risk of spreading the virus. In light of these concerns, the most pressing need was to reduce behaviors that could facilitate the transmission of Ebola. It was also of critical importance because at this stage there was still some skepticism within the community about the existence of the virus.

Community leaders took the initiative to promote specific measures aimed at ensuring the control and prevention of new infections. One of these was partnering with the CDC to learn more about the virus and what needed to be done to stop its transmission. Representatives of some Liberian immigrant groups across the United States held conference calls with the CDC, during which they were informed about specific practices they could promote to prevent the spread of Ebola. This information was shared with other Liberians, who were then asked to promote these practices when they spoke with their relatives who were still in Liberia.

It was, however, Liberian immigrant leaders who took the leading role in translating the information they received from the CDC into actionable steps that were implemented in their community. One example of this was the promotion of enhanced handwashing practices. In one Liberian church, for example, a solution of water and chlorine was placed near the entrance for use by congregants, who were encouraged to wash their hands before entering the building. It was one of several voluntary and obligatory measures used to prevent the spread of the virus in these contexts. In the church led by Bishop Roberts, the handwashing measure was coupled with additional interventions, such as the distribution of hand sanitizer among congregants. Additionally, congregants heard talks in which the bishop promoted Ebola control and the need for people returning from Liberia to be self-quarantined for twenty-one days. These quarantines were even encouraged after steps were taken at US airports to screen all travelers arriving from Africa. "I told them," he said, "that if someone comes from Liberia, even though you passed the [temperature] test,* that quarantine period, you observe it." In saying this, he was alluding to his desire to prevent the church from becoming a location where super-spreader events occurred. This point was emphasized when he added that he advised all those returning from Liberia to stay away from church until the twenty-one-day quarantine period was over. It was a strategy for preventing unintended viral transmissions that the bishop himself took very seriously. Indeed, it was one he used himself after returning from another trip he took to Liberia during the course of the epidemic.†

As the message of prevention increased, the pulpit became not just a place to proclaim the good news of the gospel but a place where pastors communicated their support for the fight against Ebola. It was not only a

---

* Trained staff from the US Department of Homeland Security's Customs and Border Protection Unit took the temperatures of all travelers arriving from Guinea, Liberia, and Sierra Leone with a noncontact thermometer. If the test showed that they had a fever, their symptoms were subsequently evaluated by a CDC quarantine station public officer to determine whether they were likely be infected with Ebola (CDC 2014).

† The first trip he took to Liberia was closer to the start of the crisis and is extensively discussed in chapter 4.

fight to protect the lives of their congregants but also a fight in which these congregants were conscripted to become preachers of the message of prevention to their families in Africa. Part of this involved using the pulpit as a platform for admonishing congregants to take practical steps such as purchasing calling cards and calling relatives in the affected countries to deliver the message of prevention. They were asked to encourage these relatives to follow preventive measures such as frequent handwashing and a refusal to interact with persons showing symptoms of an illness.

At the EIF church, Pastor Ken used this strategy to correct an error that led to the death of his aunt and cousins in Liberia. He was determined to help his surviving relatives avoid the same fate as his cousins, who contracted the virus while taking care of his aunt. What he did during these phone calls was, according to him, to "instruct the rest of my other family members back home that nobody should cross from one line to another. 'If anyone [is] sick, let the medical authorities take care of the person. You cannot bring them in. You can still save that life without putting others at risk.'"

At the church itself, he took additional steps to change normative practices that increased the risk of unintended viral transmissions. For example, he stopped the practice of asking congregants to hug first-time visitors, which was usually done to make them feel welcome. Before the outbreak, these visitors were typically required to stand and introduce themselves during worship service, after which congregants sang the church's theme song as they walked around to hug the guests. Arguing for why the change was necessary, Pastor Ken maintained that the church "didn't know who had a guest, family member, or visitor from back home" who may have traveled to Dallas with Ebola. Like Bishop Roberts, he also asked all congregants returning from visits to affected countries to stay home from church. Surprisingly, there were no objections because most of his congregants knew what was at stake. But this did not mean that the new measures were sufficient, because the social lives of his congregants continued after the end of worship services, and this exposed them to other potential sources of risk.

Take, for example, an incident that occurred during the early days of the outbreak. Pastor Ken was forced to stop a family member and another congregant from attending church services after learning of their possible exposure to the virus in a nonchurch context. The decision was informed by the events following Duncan's diagnosis, including the effort to identify people who had interacted with him before he became sick. Because the task of tracing these contacts was difficult, Pastor Ken took matters into his own hands by helping to search for such people among his congregants. In an attempt to prevent another infection, he pleaded with them to identify themselves if they had interacted with Duncan in the days following his arrival. The response he received may not have been what he expected, as he describes in the following account:

> I mean, they were tracing everything to know where [Duncan] went, who he encountered, where he passed through, and so on and so forth. . . . Some community people answered, "Yes, we were at a function with him." They tried to reach out to those people and stuff like that. There was one member [of my church] and a family member of mine who actually attended a function with him, so once I asked the question in the church and they admitted, I pulled them over and gave them a quarantine myself, that they needed to be off from church. I mean, we were abiding by rules and regulations to protect people even from themselves and to protect one another and stuff like that, so you can imagine the season that we came from.

Across the African immigrant community, there were other challenges as well. In particular, it was difficult to develop consensus around the issue of whether social events such as birthday parties and weddings should be postponed until after the outbreak. On the one hand, there were those who believed that this was necessary because of the need to promote the message of prevention. There were risks that came with attending these events because it was difficult to know which attendees had just returned from Liberia or who had interacted with an infected person visiting from the country. Therefore, the main concern was about contracting the virus through physical interaction with possibly infected persons. As one person who supported this measure explained, he knew that the virus could be transmitted by shaking hands or hugging infected people; however, he was concerned because, as he put it, "we Africans, we like to shake hands and hug people."

On the other hand, there were others who believed that it was still fine to attend social events as long as they were hosted by trusted friends within their social circles. To avoid them, they maintained, was to give in to a sense of paranoia. Restricting attendance of these events to those organized by close friends was based on an expectation of mutual trust—an implicit honor code. It was founded on reciprocal expectations of self-policing that required individuals to voluntarily stay away from social gatherings if they knew their health had been compromised. For the most part, however, these gatherings continued. However, those who attended reported noticeable changes in the tenor of these events. This time, they included short times of prayer for those affected by the epidemic and opportunities to make donations to help combat the spread of the disease.

Responding to the Needs of the Troh Family

When it came to responding to the social fallout of the local outbreak, there was no disagreement on whether the community should act. The earliest evidence of concerted action to address these consequences came after the identity of Duncan was confirmed. Shortly after Liberian immigrant leaders learned about his relationship with Troh, they became concerned by reports they received about how her family was doing while they were quarantined. The family had lost most of their belongings after their apartment was decontaminated, and there was no letup in the backlash directed toward them. Few community leaders knew the family before the outbreak, but as they learned more about them and the hardships they faced they decided to try to assist them in any way they could.

Much of the initiative demonstrated in response to the plight of the family was channeled through the CLA, because one of its core functions was to provide assistance to Liberian families in crisis. Helping the Troh family, however, brought up a number of challenges. For one, they were physically cut off from their social networks and usual sources of livelihood. In the first two days of the quarantine, the only food available to them was groceries purchased before the outbreak. When they started receiving food from a local relief organization, they discovered that some of what had been offered to them was expired (Troh 2015). And then the family had other, peculiar needs. Being quarantined kept them away from their usual sources of ethnic foods, and there were legal issues to be addressed concerning Duncan's treatment in the hospital. In addition, civic officials were doing very little to address the public stigma faced by the family. All these issues posed a serious challenge to the leaders of the CLA. Although they had responded to the crisis faced by their members in the past, they did not have the experience or resources needed to address the complex needs of the Troh family.

Given that he was one of the leaders of the CLA, George decided to call Troh while she was quarantined to see how she was doing. After that, he felt that the CLA had enough resources to help relieve some of the problems the family was facing. To start the process, he consulted other leaders to develop a strategy on how to respond. Describing the process and the issues they discussed, he said: "I called a meeting of the different officers of [our organization] to see what we [could] do to help. Louise [Troh] was then in isolation, but I was in touch with her all the time. I wanted to know what she needed, and I found out that she needed some Liberian food, clothing. She did not have anything. They were only feeding her with sandwiches, but we Africans, we need to eat our own food."

The group decided to make another call to Troh to specifically ask her for a list of things she wanted them to provide. George and a colleague then used the list to shop for the items needed to meet the family's more immediate needs. They bought her some African clothes, including a lappa,* as well as some African food, utensils, and other supplies. One problem they faced after making the purchases was the difficulty in delivering the goods to the family. They were leery of leading journalists to the place where the family was quarantined, so they took the supplies to a local center that was in contact with the family for onward transmission to Troh.

This response was notable for several reasons. First, it was a clear demonstration of agency by Liberian immigrants to act to address the culturally specific needs of the family. It showed their unwillingness to stand by and watch as one of their own experienced a period of misfortune. Second, the response was instructive for capturing the implied limits they faced in their attempts to meet the needs of the family. While they could provide for the family's most immediate needs, there was nothing they could do to protect them from the intense backlash they received from the public. Furthermore, they were limited in their ability to meet other needs, such

---

* A lappa is a large colorful wrapper that is worn by men and women in West Africa. Women typically tie it around their waist and sometimes wear it informally in the house.

as finding a permanent home for the family at the end of the quarantine. Addressing these issues required the intervention of complementary institutions from outside their community.

Local political leadership for tempering the stigma faced by the Troh family was provided by Clay Jenkins. A prominent judge in Dallas County, he took several public steps to counter the backlash faced by the family and the widespread misinformation about the nature of the virus. One of the first things he did was advocate for a response to the outbreak based on science, not fear. Accordingly, he gave multiple press briefings in which he repeatedly pointed out that the virus could not be transmitted unless one makes contact with the bodily fluids of someone showing symptoms of the disease (Weiss 2014). As if to make this point clear, he visited Troh's apartment without wearing any protective equipment, in full view of journalists. Later on, he put the family in his vehicle and took them speeding past reporters on their way to the secret location where their quarantine was completed (Troh 2015).

Related to this was a response that involved a collaboration between African immigrant leaders and the civil rights leader Reverend Jesse Jackson. Concerns had been expressed in some sections of the community that Africans lacked the strong political voice needed to shift the public narrative on Duncan's experiences. Working with Jackson was seen as one way to fill this void. However, there were others who were worried that he might ask the community to conduct a public protest, which was not something its leaders were open to doing. Collaborating with Reverend Jackson, however, was a way of using the shared ancestral connections between Africans and African Americans as a source of social capital needed to meet a community objective. Compared to African immigrants, who "did not have a voice," as one immigrant leader reasoned, African Americans were "the most powerful" Black people on earth and had a history of supporting humanitarian and political causes in Africa.*

Whether Reverend Jackson's presence changed public perceptions toward African immigrants in Dallas remains unclear. What is clear is that

---

* This immigrant leader was referring to Martin Luther King Jr.'s support for the African leaders in their struggle for independence and the subsequent efforts of African Amer-

during his brief presence in the city, he joined African immigrant leaders in a public prayer for Duncan at the THP hospital. This was followed by a press conference, during which he asked for compassion to be extended toward Duncan while drawing attention to the possible role of race in influencing the hospital's initial reaction to the patient. To many African immigrants, this display of solidarity was seen to have affected the subsequent actions taken by the THP hospital. Following this news conference, the hospital established a foundation to support public health in Liberia. This, some immigrant leaders believed, would not have happened without the support Reverend Jackson provided.

In terms of taking care of the Troh family at the end of their quarantine, there was very little the community could do. Once again, complementary support was provided from outside the community to make this possible. This help came from the Wilshire Baptist Church, the church Troh attended, and its intervention in the crisis was peculiar. For one, Troh's association with the church started after she decided to fellowship with them rather than other African churches in the city because of what they did for her two nieces. Members of the church's Sunday school class had provided services to them as part of their outreach to refugees in the city. As a result, when her nieces invited her to the church, she decided to attend and continued to do so regularly thereafter. The church's intervention was also unusual because its members were predominantly White and elderly. Therefore, their decision to intervene was one that crossed racial lines and was inconsistent with the notion that elderly Whites would refuse to provide assistance to racial minorities as the United States becomes more diverse (Lichter 2013).

Susan, who helped the Troh family search for an apartment,* was the church member in charge of the family's postquarantine reintegration. Describing the specifics of how the church helped the Troh family, Susan started by highlighting how their lead pastor became concerned about the plight of Troh after learning about her connection to Duncan. This con-

ican political leaders to push for US sanctions against South Africa during the period of apartheid.
* This was discussed in the previous chapter.

cern led him to join Judge Jenkins on his daily visits to the family while they were quarantined. Apart from this, the church helped to replace some of the personal items destroyed in Troh's apartment. Using donations they received on Troh's behalf, they also helped pay her bills after she lost her job as a result of the stigma of Ebola.

As the following account given by Susan indicates, the assistance the church provided during this process focused on meeting the family's practical needs in ways that few institutions were equipped to do at the time.

> What people sent in to give, we kept a real accurate account of that, so that she knew what was being done with it. And we bought her lots of gift cards for groceries. I took her shopping once to the Hong Kong Market, which was fun, to get to see, like, what do you actually need? Because a Tom Thumb Grocery is okay, but you need food that you like, and so we did that, and . . . we took her car down and got that fixed. We had a great mechanic who did it for quite a discount. So . . . it was really a community-wide response where people, not just Wilshire but different organizations and different good-natured, good-hearted people, said, "Yeah, we'll help for sure."

Part of this community-wide response involved collaborating with Liberian immigrant organizations to conduct a memorial service for Duncan after his death. The service was designed according to the wishes of Troh; however, Liberian immigrant leaders were asked to play an active role in the event—in part because of the need to involve members of the community who were most affected by the crisis. About 250 people attended the memorial service, most of whom were visiting the church for the first time. All told, this intervention by the church was an important display of how outside institutions stepped in to support what was started by African immigrant organizations to address the fallout of the outbreak.

Confronting the Stigma of Ebola

Supporting the needs of the Troh family was only part of the general response of African immigrants to the consequences of the outbreak. Of equal concern was the need to address the stigma of Ebola directed toward the community. Confronting this issue required action to be taken by individuals and by immigrant organizations. In both cases, there was enough evidence to underscore the significance of agency for mitigating the effect of the backlash. This task required addressing stigmas encountered in various social contexts and was pursued using three strategies. The first was the use of false or alternative African identities; the second, the threat of legal action; and the third, public education.

The use of alternative African identities was the most common method employed for dealing with encounters of stigma. Its basic premise was choosing when to claim or conceal specific African national identities as a way to shift public attention away from immigrants from Ebola-affected countries. At its core, the strategy exploited the widespread ignorance of African geography and the public's inability to distinguish between people from different African groups. The reason it was attractive was clear. It shifted control over encounters with stigma from the hands of the public to those of stigmatized individuals. In so doing, it gave the latter the power to redirect the course of social interactions that made them vulnerable to acts of prejudice.

In practice, the strategy involved claiming the national identities of African countries far from the source of the epidemic. This was done as a way to preempt the concerns of locals who were afraid to interact with immigrants from West Africa. A key assumption of the strategy was that locals specifically associated the threat of the virus with immigrants from Liberia, and to some extent Sierra Leone and Guinea. By claiming to be from Zimbabwe rather than from Liberia, for example, one could attempt to decrease the likelihood of being stigmatized. This temporary rejection of these identities had the instrumental purpose of allowing African immigrants to live some semblance of a normal life. As Cosmas, who was from Kenya, explained, the use of this strategy by his African peers made sense because "you don't want to stand out in the crowd." It was not the first time he had seen Africans in the city conceal their identities in this way. The first time he saw it being used was among Rwandan refugees who arrived in Dallas in the 1990s. Many of them claimed they were from Burundi when asked about their origins in order to avoid being associated with the genocide in Rwanda.

However, when Paul discussed why he and other Liberians employed this approach, he focused on two additional reasons. The first was their fear of the unknown, and it was linked with their belief that the hostile response directed toward Liberians would have the same tragic consequences for them as it did for Japanese immigrants during World War II. Explaining his view further, he said: "Everyone was afraid because in America, a long time ago, when America was fighting a war with Japan, they took all the Japanese and put them all in a concentration camp. So can you imagine what they would do now that a Liberian had come to the country with Ebola? Liberians in Dallas were scared. Before, anytime there was an event like a funeral of a Liberian, everyone would go to the funeral. But when the Ebola crisis happened, it was a mess. Everyone was scared."

He further gave an example of how the strategy of using alternative African identities worked. "One Liberian I know," he said, "a guy named [Jeff], when he was asked whether he was from Liberia, he said no, he was from Cameroon [laughs]." The best comparison that Paul could think of was an incident described in the Bible. "You remember when they say Peter denied Christ?" he asked rhetorically, "He said no, I don't know the man."

A second reason Paul gave for using this strategy was the need to counter the economic effects of stigma. Rumors and stories of actual experiences with stigma were so pervasive that most people in the Liberian community had heard about how it was negatively affecting African-owned businesses. Given that he was the owner of a convenience store, Paul assumed that knowledge of his national identity would have a similar effect on his business. To avoid this, he chose to conceal his Liberian identity. Describing his interactions with customers during this period, he said: "People used to come here and say, 'Are you guys Liberian?' We would say no. Even though we are from Liberia, when we were doing business with them we told them no." In the end, the strategy worked as Paul had expected.

For businesses such as hair-braiding salons and African restaurants, which were built around the provision of culturally specific products, it was less effective. In Minnesota, for example, a Liberian restaurant owner changed the name of her restaurant from Mama Ti's African Kitchen to Mama Ti's Kitchen and Deli to distance herself from Africa after experiencing a decline in patronage during the crisis (Goodnough 2014). However, the stigma she faced was so strong that the change had no effect in reversing the decline in her business.

Compared to this somewhat evasive strategy, the pursuit of possible legal action was a direct approach used to fight stigma. Faced with increasing reports of discrimination against their members, Liberian immigrants organized a meeting to develop a concerted strategy to address the issue. Anyone who had been sent home from work or who had children who experienced discrimination at school because they were Liberian was instructed to report it to them. Their intention was, as George put it, "to take [the reports] to the proper authorities because discrimination is illegal." It was also a strategy that was consistent with the Department of Justice's general warning to federal workers to guard against the likelihood of discrimination against Africans based on their perceived association with the virus (Delaney 2014).

Another direct approach was to be proactive by educating the public about Ebola and Africa as a way of preempting encounters with stigma. This approach was important for several reasons. First, it was a less confrontational strategy that could be used by individuals as well as institutions. Second, it represented a coordinated effort to correct misinformation about how the virus is transmitted. Such corrective efforts included one developed by Sierra Leonean immigrant organizations, which decided to engage the public in formal discussions about various aspects of the ongoing crisis. It was implemented in the form of a seminar at a major hotel in Dallas, to which the public and members of the media were invited to learn about the virus and its relationship to the African community. Lans, a Sierra Leonean academic and long-term resident of the area, was one of the speakers at the event. From his perspective, the event helped his organization achieve several objectives, including increasing awareness of the diversity of the West African immigrant community in the city, underscoring the fact that not every African in the United States was affected by the disease, and helping them make modest steps toward changing the narrative that all West Africans were infected with Ebola. Although these objectives were laudable, the event did not receive the level of coverage the organization had hoped to achieve, since most of its attendees were Africans themselves and not other local residents. This was probably because the same fears and stigmas that the organizers were trying to combat were the same fears that kept locals from attending the event.

At the individual level, the goal of public education was more modest. It simply involved using encounters with stigma as teaching opportunities to educate Americans about Africa's diversity and to dispel myths about Ebola. This was what Nancy was trying to do after returning from Sierra Leone during the epidemic and realizing that some of her friends were afraid to interact with her. Rather than being flustered by the reactions, she used their concerns as an opportunity

> to educate people because, for example, people will say, "Oh, you know [Nancy] is from Sierra Leone, where this was going on." And I'd say, "Yes, but I have been here twenty-one days." But sometimes if I want to tease them I'll say, "I've been here less than twenty-one days." You know, and they'll look at me funny because they know I'm joking, and I've been around here. But I use it to educate them because they talk as if it's everyone in the country that has Ebola, everybody is poor, there is nobody that's walking around that's healthy, so I use it to educate them about Africa and about Sierra Leone specifically.

Nevertheless, confronting the stigma was not without its challenges. Among the most important was that it did not involve the same degree of coordination between African groups affected in Dallas as that seen elsewhere in the country. In Minnesota, for example, African immigrants formed the Minnesota African Task Force against Ebola, which was considered the largest community-based response to the Ebola outbreak in the United States (Almendrala 2015). The task force's strategy was diverse. It formed an Ebola stigma legal response team to deal with the surge in prejudice against Africans and, as was the case among Liberian immigrants in Dallas, explored legal options available for dealing with experiences of discrimination (Almendrala 2015). The group also provided public education to members of its own community to warn them about the dangers of visiting the affected West African countries during the crisis. Furthermore, it lobbied the state's representatives to vote for the emergency Ebola funding request in Congress and to advocate for temporary protected status for immigrants from Guinea, Liberia, and Sierra Leone.* This effort capped their attempts to deal with the consequences of the outbreak in their own context.

---

* Temporary protected status is a temporary immigration status given to nationals of countries affected by short-term crises such as hurricanes and other natural disasters, and in some cases armed conflict.

Immigrant Institutions and the International Response

Compared to the local response to the outbreak's fallout, the international response to the epidemic differed. For one, the former was largely defensive in nature and focused on combating the immediate threat of the outbreak and its consequences for individuals. By contrast, the international response was more proactive. Part of this was because, with the exception of the few people who lost loved ones to the virus in West Africa, much of the fallout of the epidemic in the region was felt vicariously. Another difference between the two was that the international response required taking actions that were less likely to involve physical contact between locals and African immigrants, such as sending donations. Even more important was the level of urgency associated with the international response relative to the local one. More Ebola fatalities were being recorded in affected countries in West Africa than in Dallas, and it soon became clear that institutions in these countries were less equipped to deal with the consequences of the epidemic compared to those in Dallas. In light of these realities, the primary objective of the international response was to provide assistance to health institutions in affected countries.

It was an objective that benefited from the high degree of altruism within the community as well as a desire among local institutions to help countries affected by the outbreak. As a result, it was easy to develop partnerships in the city that crossed social and cultural lines. For example, it was easier for immigrants from affected West African countries to collaborate with immigrants from other parts of Africa as well as with local businesses and churches. Altruism was also a key factor that made it easy to overcome the inertia created by concerns about what would happen to the financial assistance that was sent to governments in Africa. Skeptics were apprehensive of whether their donations would reach the right people. However, as one African immigrant leader observed, his response was to let them know that while their concern was legitimate, it was still important for them to do "what God had placed in [their] hearts to do and [not] worry about the rest."

Successfully mounting a meaningful international response meant exploiting the strengths of ethnic institutions in the African immigrant community. One of these strengths was their existing infrastructure for conducting transnational humanitarian activities between Dallas and West Africa. They had developed systems to transfer food, used clothing, and other resources to the region to provide relief to the poor. Within the community, there were also diverse organizations within national immigrant groups that had a well-developed history of collaboration. In particular, both Liberian and Sierra Leonean immigrants had national umbrella organizations with established links with ethnic organizations in their communities. These links provided the critical foundation for initiating and coordinating the response to the epidemic in West Africa.

For example, when Ralph, a leader in the Organization of Sierra Leoneans in Texas, described the origins of their effort to respond to the Ebola crisis in Sierra Leone, his account revealed that they were simply leveraging their prior experience of working together. Providing the background on how this response was developed, he said:

> We had been meeting, organizing events in the community, and people were being very supportive. And every time, all the organizations made contributions [to these events], and we did these things, so now, when there was this outbreak of Ebola, we already had the foundation. We already had the structure, so we encouraged other organizations to send representatives on the [conference] call as we went ahead and planned, so that was the main strategy, so it was very easy for the other organizations to send representatives—one or two representatives—and to come on the conference call as we worked on the modality of how we could be of help.

Among Liberian immigrants, the story was familiar. They had a similar history of developing collaborative relationships to address common problems, and in the past they used these relationships to respond to the humanitarian crisis created by their country's civil war. Given this history, the task of developing an international response simply involved scaling up these patterns of collaboration and exploiting the strength of the infrastructure found in more established ethnic institutions. In this case, these institutions were mainly members of the network of Liberian churches scattered across the Dallas metropolitan area.

Because the main objective of the international response was to support healthcare institutions in the affected countries, it was important to secure access to several types of resources to make it possible. The most accessible of these were found among African immigrants themselves. Since the level of resources needed was substantial, existing traditions of fund-raising established by ethnic organizations proved to be useful, but they needed to be complemented by other approaches as well. Small-scale efforts by organizations such as the Mandingo cultural association were thus expanded to include a greater level of collaboration between groups. Indeed, this period marked one of the few times that such a diverse collection of organizations, such as churches, alumni associations of schools in West Africa, professional organizations, and sports teams, collaborated to raise funds for the same purpose.

Within each organization, the easiest method used to raise funds was to ask members to make specific monetary contributions. These contributions were either transferred to pan-national immigrant organizations, such as the CLA, or used to purchase relief supplies that were then sent to affected countries. In immigrant churches, fund-raising efforts involved collecting monetary contributions other than those collected from regular donations during services. Funds were also raised by ethnic organizations associated with Africans from countries other than those at the center of the outbreak. These included funds collected by Nigerian ethnic churches and other Africans in the community who wanted to show solidarity with their counterparts during their time of need.

The overall institutional response further required a search for more diverse types of contributions. Of critical importance was the need for human resources. Labor was required to reach out to possible donors outside the African community, coordinate the overall campaign, and perform manual tasks such as packing donations into shipping containers before they were transported to West Africa. The labor needed to complete these activities was provided almost exclusively by volunteers within the African community, and it represented an alternative way of contributing to the global effort for those with limited access to other types of resources.

Beyond these efforts, African immigrants tapped into their social networks in the wider Dallas community to secure additional resources. Long-term immigrants had well-developed ties to networks in the city, which enabled them to tap into new sources of financial and material resources. Unlike their counterparts, who were either in the working class or were otherwise disadvantaged, these immigrants included business executives, medical doctors, teachers, and members the professional class, many of whom had lived in the city for a decade and beyond. They not only had resources of their own but also knew people in strategic places who could connect them with the resources they needed. Notwithstanding the widespread fear of African immigrants, there was enough goodwill among many Dallas residents to support the international campaign. It was easy to see the need for doing something to address the source of the epidemic in West Africa because failing to act had the risk of generating further negative consequences for people in the city.

The goodwill found within these networks was central to Josiah's quest to find resources for the response to the epidemic in Sierra Leone. As such, the main group he used to access these resources was his large network of American friends. Starting the process was relatively simple. He handed out flyers to friends at his place of work, requesting help getting access to donated hospital equipment. Next, he turned to friends at the mainstream church he attended, who directly and indirectly provided the bulk of what he collected. While the solicitation process started very simply, it morphed into a progressive series of movements between referral steps that led him from one source of resources to another. The best example of this was seen in his description of the process that led him to an organization that donated hospital beds to his cause:

> I called a friend of mine who I've known for a long time; we both serve in church, and we still stay connected. She referred me to another friend who was working for [a relief organization]. . . . Being a Christian organization, they have a program for charity—on how to help countries, churches, and hospitals around the world. This friend, she was not working for [the organization] anymore, but she told me, she said, "[Josiah], I know a friend who is directly involved with similar programs and might be able to help with hospital beds, supplies, and whatever you guys will need to be able to help with the Ebola crisis." I said, "Sure," so she gave me the contact and I called them.

Through this process of referral, the organization at the final point of the referral chain invited Josiah to their warehouse to select various types of hospital equipment. They further offered to pack the equipment in a shipping container. The only thing he was required to do was pay for the cost of shipping the container to West Africa.

Other organizations used a more structured approach to tap into the wealth of resources found within the larger Dallas community. For example, the Krio ethnic organization in Dallas developed a strategy of targeting specific institutions such as hospitals for donated medical supplies and other equipment. Recalling their message to these institutions, Tayo, one of the organization's leaders, said it was simply "whatever you have—excess supplies, essential things that would help with the epidemic—and if you don't have anything, you can make a monetary donation. We could use that too." This was not just a casual attempt to get institutions to donate. It involved a formal process that was carefully planned and executed. Members of the organization were provided with official letters that they could use to request these resources, and the origin of these letters had a story of its own. Specifically, Tayo used his relationship with the Sierra Leonean ambassador in Washington, DC, to arrange for the letters to be written on the official letterhead of the embassy, which would provide an added sense of authenticity. Describing the strategy used in their overall enterprise, he maintained that they "sent people to go talk to their churches, their places of employment, and the like. I usually backed them up with a letter from the embassy just to let people know that what they were doing was legitimate. I had the ambassador write several letters for me and send them to me. I asked him to write it to the company we are requesting help from, and to just cc me so I could follow up with whoever they were writing to."

To complement this endeavor, Tayo tapped into his own personal networks to secure other types of resources. Near where his business is located was an organization that specialized in the provision of medical assistance to developing countries. He used his relationship with the director to get two additional types of assistance. First, he secured their help in purchasing and shipping medical equipment to Sierra Leone. Second, he successfully appealed to them to promote his cause with companies such as Shell and Chevron, which were among the major clients of the organization. Overall, the strategy paid off—and in a big way. Tayo received a large stock of supplies such as medical gloves, personal protective equipment, and donations from local food banks, as well as financial contributions, which he used to ship the supplies. Indeed, the supplies were so extensive that it took seven large shipping containers to ship them to Sierra Leone.

Other individuals had similar local connections that they used to request assistance to ship donated supplies to West Africa. One such individual was Lans, who had a well-developed relationship with a church organization close to his place of work. It was a well-funded Baptist organization that he had persuaded to provide humanitarian services to poor communities in his native Sierra Leone before the epidemic. Because of this venture, the organization had a long track record of providing services to orphans and poor farmers in the country. When Lans approached them this time to see if they would help transport medical supplies to West Africa, they agreed. They offered to provide shipping container space that could be used to transfer donated supplies from Dallas to Ebola hot spots in the region.

Apart from these structured attempts to utilize local social capital, there were other opportunities to support the international response that appeared to be serendipitous. It turned out, for example, that Kent Brantly, the American doctor who had been infected with the disease in Liberia, had strong ties to the city of Dallas. After the outbreak in the city, he was willing to assist the Liberian community in their efforts to fight the epidemic in the country. Leaders of these immigrants then collaborated with him to organize a fund-raising event that was also attended by a representative of the CDC. During the event, Brantly gave a speech to attendees and helped raise approximately $10,000 for Ebola control efforts in Liberia. These funds were used to purchase medical supplies (e.g., personal protective equipment) that were sent to treat Ebola-infected patients in the country.

As media coverage of the crisis increased, there were also unexpected inflows of resources to support the campaign against the epidemic in West Africa. Representatives of church organizations, businesses, and other mainstream institutions in Dallas sought out immigrant leaders, offering various types of assistance needed to help affected communities in Africa. These offers came from organizations such as Bank of America, the Lutheran Church, and the Texas Baptist Convention. Additionally, several Dallas-based companies developed systems that allowed their employees to make voluntary financial contributions to the fight against the epidemic.

Most of these funds were offered to Liberian immigrant organizations and were used in the effort to support healthcare institutions in the country.

As expected, the effort to raise local resources was not without its challenges. One challenge was the risk of duplication because many African immigrants were members of multiple ethnic organizations. Added to this was the fact that some of these organizations were targeting the same set of donors within the city. Of these two, however, the challenge of multiple organization membership was easier to address. Because monetary donations were not obligatory, immigrants had the option of donating to one and not to another. It was also theoretically possible for them to donate different types of resources between organizations, such as donating money to one organization and labor to another. Targeting the same pool of donors was a problem but less so when donors were open to providing assistance to multiple immigrant groups. In some cases, however, there was a specific desire among donors to contribute to the international response in Liberia, and this was possibly because news coverage of the local outbreak was mainly tied to the Liberian immigrant community.

Executing the International Response

On the other side of the Atlantic, the international response initiated in Dallas benefited from African immigrants' ability to leverage the advantages of transnational social capital. As shown in previous studies, transnational migrants' interactions between origin and destination societies place them within global networks that give them access to unique types of capital, which can be deployed across space (Faist 2008). This capital can be used to provide loans to family members in origin countries or to pay for the resources needed to meet the start-up costs of entrepreneurs (Katila and Wahlbeck 2012). More frequently, however, immigrants use transnational social capital to operate as agents of development. In other words, their embeddedness in transnational networks allows them to transmit resources across borders to improve the lives of the marginalized in less developed countries (Faist 2008). Much of what was done in terms of implementing the goals of the international response to the epidemic was in line with this role of immigrants as agents of development. In this case, however, the primary focus of this role was to support the weak health systems that had become overburdened by the task of combating the spread of the virus in West Africa.

Local networks in the region played a critical role in laying the groundwork for implementing the response. In the early stages of this process, they were used to identify areas of priority that immigrants in Dallas could use to fine-tune their fund-raising efforts. Networks within government offices in countries affected by the epidemic were used to identify the specific needs of healthcare institutions leading the fight against Ebola, and these needs were used in several ways. Among Sierra Leonean immigrants, for example, the funds raised during their campaign were only used to purchase supplies for the country that were identified as necessities by their local contacts. As a Sierra Leonean immigrant recalled, these local contacts "kind of took the lead and were giving us directions as to what would work." The needs identified by local contacts were also used in the process of soliciting specific types of donations in Dallas. Government officials in Sierra Leone were asked to provide a list of the supplies most needed by local hospitals, and their list was used to request donations of specific types of medical equipment and supplies from Dallas hospitals.

Where transnational networks were most important was in using resources sent from Dallas to fund specific types of programs. One example of this involved the use of funds raised among immigrants in Dallas by officials in Sierra Leone, who collaborated with them to conduct a public health campaign. One of these immigrants knew the director of a TV station in the country who used his influence to secure the assistance of his employer to promote the campaign. After this was secured, the partnership between the immigrant donors in Dallas and their local partners in Sierra Leone became operational. To get the ball rolling, the donors sent about $5,000 to their local partners, after which the latter went to work printing flyers that were distributed at markets in Freetown as part of an effort to sensitize residents of the city about the threat of Ebola. The overall message of the campaign was one that emphasized the importance of disease prevention through actions such as limiting contact with bodily fluids and allowing health workers rather than family members to handle the burial of corpses.

Another common strategy for utilizing transnational social capital involved leveraging established organizations that sent assistance to the affected countries before the start of the epidemic to address new issues. This required many African immigrant organizations in Dallas to refocus their operations to target the health needs of Ebola-affected communities and expand their fund-raising activities to support the new needs created by the epidemic. This was the strategy used by the Mandingo cultural association in Dallas to respond to the epidemic in Liberia. Prior to this, their main approach for providing transnational humanitarian assistance was to conduct biannual trips to the country in order to serve poor communities. However, when they learned from their local contacts that there was a lack of ambulances to transport sick Ebola patients to hospitals, they decided to refocus their attention to address this challenge. Various chapters of the association around Texas raised funds to make this possible. The Dallas chapter raised about $7,000, and the chapter based in Houston raised about $8,000. These funds were pooled with contributions from other chapters to successfully purchase the vehicle. Speaking with pride as he explained the significance of their accomplishment, Alim, a leader in the group, maintained that "there was no car to transport the people, and Ebola is a very fast-moving disease, so now when somebody had problems, the car would go faster and take them to the hospital."

There is no question that providing this type of material assistance was important. However, there were other challenges created by the epidemic in West Africa that required the development of more innovative responses. This was seen in an attempt to provide sustenance to healthcare workers affected by the consequences of the outbreak in Sierra Leone by immigrants from the country who were part of a specific transnational social network. The group in question was an organization of Sierra Leonean nurses abroad who had made annual visits to the country to provide humanitarian assistance prior to the epidemic. As the epidemic spread throughout the country, they learned about the negative ways in which it was affecting a small village clinic that they usually worked with during their visits. It was located in an area where new Ebola cases were increasing, and as a result the government had ordered it to shut down its operations. This decision was taken as a precaution. The government wanted to channel the treatment of Ebola patients from small clinics such as this one to larger healthcare facilities with better-trained employees who could handle the disease. However, the order created inadvertent problems for the clinic's employees. Because payments received from patients were the main source of income used for salaries, complying with the order would have eliminated a major source of their livelihood. Therefore, rather than completely shutting down, the clinic's employees planned to scale back operations to allow the inflow of funds to help them pay their bills.

In Dallas, Nancy was concerned when she learned about these plans during her communications with the small village clinic. As a healthcare worker, she understood the dangers of having untrained workers treat patients who were potentially infected with the virus. Consequently, she expressed her disagreement with the plan but knew more should be done to encourage them to comply. What followed was a show of agency that went beyond the usual work between her group and the clinic. When describing the actions she took, she observed the following:

> I said [to them], "I don't think so. Please shut down. I am going to find a way." ... And I didn't know how I was going to find it, "but I'm going to find a way" ... because it's a staff of like 10. It's a small community clinic, including the cleaner, everyone else, so we said, "We're going to support them so they can pay their bills." So we paid salaries for them for six months. So friends would give money. People would donate. We even had a friend who did a prayer breakfast to raise funds for them.

This action was instructive because it also spoke to the broader consequences of the outbreak on the livelihoods of those in the affected countries. Transnational networks became a viable tool for addressing these consequences, especially when they affected the welfare of the relatives of immigrants in Dallas. The growing epidemic caused more of them to stay home from work due to the closure of government offices and some private businesses. Consequently, the responsibility of providing for the needs of these relatives fell into the hands of their more fortunate kinsmen in Dallas.

Meeting these responsibilities required taking action in Dallas to find additional sources of income. The most frequent way this was done was by taking a second job, and the practice was so prevalent that it negatively affected attendance at community events. Besides these community effects, it also had negative consequences for physical and mental health. For example, according to Manneh, a member of one of the immigrant soccer teams, the new responsibilities had an emotional toll on him and his team members. Describing this toll, he said: "A lot of guys were stressed physically, and mentally, [and] they weren't [at practices] because everybody had to get a part-time job or work extra hours just to send money back home." However, the inconvenience of working extra hours paled in comparison to the consequences of having their relatives in West Africa putting themselves in harm's way. Fortunately, many of them were able to avoid these consequences as a result of the embeddedness of their kinsmen in transnational family networks.

Understanding Why the Immigrant Response to the Crisis Matters

To put these responses in perspective, it is important to remember that African immigrants faced the brunt of the negative consequences of the Ebola outbreak in Dallas. However, during this period they were not paralyzed by fear of the virus in their community nor by concerns about the spread of the disease in West Africa. Despite having regular encounters with stigma and being at the center of the narrative of blame, they found ways to take action geared toward mitigating the fallout of the crisis. All the evidence on the actions they took supports the conclusion that they failed to yield to the tendency of merely seeing themselves as victims. Instead, these immigrants took intentional actions and developed prosocial initiatives to improve their welfare as well as that of communities in African countries affected by the epidemic. This is not to say that their actions forestalled the effects of the backlash they faced during this period. Rather, it is to recognize that in the face of these challenges, they knew how to use their institutions and resources to develop counteractions to address the negative consequences of the outbreak on both sides of the Atlantic. These actions provide us with several lessons on community responses to epidemics.

We learn from the response to the local outbreak, for example, that immigrants are just as committed to using control measures that prevent the spread of disease as native-born populations. While this should be intuitive, it runs counter to the tendency of societies experiencing epidemics to specifically link immigrants with the spread of disease. African immigrants' commitment to disease control was an acknowledgment of the highly contagious nature of the virus and the fact that it threatened lives in their community as much as it did on the outside. Their response demonstrated that they were not bogged down by the debate on who should be blamed for the spread of the virus in the city. Although it was important for them to challenge the dominant narrative of blame, the need to prevent more Ebola transmissions was too urgent for them not to take action. In light of these realities, they took steps to promote positive health behaviors such as handwashing with a chlorine solution and enforced measures such as personal quarantines in an attempt to keep their communities safe from the virus. Despite the fact that they lacked the training of community health workers, they showed their agency in recognizing the risk posed by the virus and developing contextualized responses to foster the use of good health practices in the community.

Their response to the social fallout of the outbreak further illustrates their use of agency to change the course of their interactions with the public. Whether it was through the use of alternative ethnic identities, the threat of lawsuits, or engagement with the public, they took actions that showed that the stigma of disease does not always remain unchallenged by the stigmatized. There was no question about what these actions were trying to achieve. As a form of social resistance, they were pushing back—they were fighting against the forces that threatened their community. This resistance, however, started much earlier in the outbreak. When critics promoted a narrative of blame, they fought to discredit the narrative and develop one of their own. Subsequently, the use of African identities to classify themselves as targets of stigma led them to organize themselves to take appropriate action against the sources of stigma. These actions did not reverse the dominant narrative of blame, but they had a fair degree of success at the personal level. Although the morality of using alternative identities could be debated, it was at this level that these immigrants were most able to shift the course of social interactions that were likely to make them targets of stigma.

From their international response to the epidemic in West Africa, we also learn that the agency of immigrants in responding to the crisis is not restricted by constraints of national boundaries. In one sense, their efforts to send resources to affected countries in the region were similar to those of diaspora populations that promote economic development ventures in their homelands (Mercer et al. 2013; Wei and Balasubramanyam 2006).

However, the international response of Africans in Dallas was also significant in two important ways. The first was in its objective—it was specifically focused on saving lives affected by an unprecedented global health emergency. As a result, it focused on the transfer of financial and material resources to support health institutions abroad. The second was in the diverse contributions that were used to mount the response. They involved the use of a rare combination of financial resources, material donations, and religious activities, all in an effort to confront the threat of disease in less developed countries.

Similarly, we learn that this international response did not just benefit from the resources found within the African immigrant community. It depended on the utilization of local sources of social capital found elsewhere in Dallas, as well as on active partnerships between African immigrants and native-born citizens. These collaborations illustrate the need for more clarity in how the role of the latter is represented in the discourse of epidemics tied to immigrants. In many cases, they are mainly conceptualized as the sources of stigma. However, as the experiences of African immigrants indicate, native-born populations can also be actively involved in partnerships with immigrants to fight against the negative consequences of public health emergencies.

In the same vein, the execution of the international response developed in the African community in Dallas could not have been successful without the use of transnational social capital. As the evidence presented indicates, residents of Liberia and Sierra Leone were more than just recipients of the resources they received from immigrants in Dallas. Occasionally, they contributed to the response by providing information used to fine-tune the accumulation of resources and for implementing public health programs in West Africa. In other words, the success of the international response to the epidemic was a consequence of the combined influence of local partners in Africa as well institutions and individuals found both within and outside of the African immigrant community. This combination is instructive because it demonstrates an important dimension of contemporary globalization processes. That is, these processes now enable grassroots organizations to collaborate across contexts in ways that help them more effectively tackle the fallout of global humanitarian crises.

8 Conclusion

On August 1, 2018, the government of the Democratic Republic of Congo announced that four new cases of Ebola had been found in the country. The new cases were discovered after tests were conducted on samples collected in the North Kivu region. A week prior to this, the DRC had proclaimed the end of an earlier Ebola outbreak in a region more than a thousand miles from North Kivu (WHO 2018). The more recent outbreak started with the death of a sixty-five-year-old woman, after which seven of her relatives tested positive for the virus (Matthews 2018). Despite the development of new treatments for Ebola following the 2014 West African epidemic, by the end of August 2018 at least forty-seven people died from the disease in North Kivu (Matthews 2018). This is concerning, especially given that the outbreak occurred in a region located along the country's border with three countries: Burundi, Rwanda, and Uganda. Furthermore, North Kivu is a region with a recent history of armed conflict. As a result, it is the source of frequent migrations from the DRC and its neighboring countries.

The start of the outbreak in North Kivu three years after the end of the epidemic in West Africa reminded us of the continued existence of Ebola. When the outbreak occurred in North Kivu, it marked the tenth time that the DRC had experienced an Ebola crisis following the first outbreak, which was documented in 1976 near the Ebola River (Matthews 2018). The North Kivu outbreak was also a reminder that, at least in the short term, very little had changed in the determinants of the spread of the virus. As in previous epidemics, one of the most important of these was migration. To respond to concerns about the spread of Ebola from North Kivu, relief organizations deployed epidemiologists, medical doctors, and other professionals to help with disease surveillance at various points along the DRC's borders (IOM 2018). In neighboring Uganda, migrants arriving from North Kivu were required to have their temperatures taken and to step into tubs filled with chlorinated water in order to disinfect their shoes (Sun and Bernstein 2018).

Since the end of the West African epidemic, the United States has not experienced such a direct threat of Ebola transmission through migration. Yet, with continued outbreaks of diseases abroad and given the centrality of migration to contemporary globalization processes, the country remains vulnerable to such threats in the future. These threats have been found in the gradual increase in the number of global epidemics as well as in the sources of infectious diseases of concern over the past three decades (Smith et al. 2014). Besides outbreaks of Ebola in Africa, more recent threats to global health have included outbreaks of chikungunya in Italy, MERS-CoV in Saudi Arabia, Diphtheria–Cox in Bangladesh, and the avian flu in China (WHO 2017a; 2017b; 2017c; 2017d). Whether future global epidemics will have the same effect on American society as that of the 2014 Ebola epidemic remains unknown. However, we can prepare for these consequences by paying attention to the key lessons we learned from this experience.

Global migration is likely to continue to be a critical determinant of the spread of epidemics and an influence on the ways in which American communities respond to these events. Moreover, the influence of these migrations will be observed on several levels. Across US metropolitan areas, it will continue to lead to the growth of new immigrant settlements. As shown in the African immigrant experience, however, the significance of migration will not just be linked to its effect on the arrival of new immigrants but will extend to the development of viable immigrant communities and to increases in racial and ethnic diversity in these settlements. Unlike ethnic communities formed by singular groups such as Mexican or Chinese immigrants, new communities will include people from more diverse national groups and represent new forms of cultural expression. In general, this diversity will be an important source of strength; however, it will also increase the availability of cultural symbols that could be used to develop stereotypes for racializing immigrants during periods of crisis.

Apart from this, globalization processes will continue to have more direct influences on societies, which could shape the course of epidemics. Through their influence on transnational connections, for example, they could increase the circumstances by which immigrants are exposed to new infectious diseases abroad. The presence of these connections between Dallas and West Africa represented a key mechanism for exposing immigrants to the potential risk of Ebola infection during their visits to the latter. Fortunately, these risks were never connected to an Ebola diagnosis among African immigrants. In other contexts, however, these connections could lead to unintended disease transmissions across international borders. Small-scale representations of these connections were among the principal factors responsible for the spread of Ebola among West African border communities. Compared to the circulatory transnational movements that originated in Dallas, these migrations occurred over shorter distances, were more frequent, and involved larger numbers of people. More importantly, they illustrated the ways in which infectious disease can be transmitted between countries in the absence of proper protocols of disease surveillance.

Transnational migration will also continue to be important for increasing awareness about the consequences of epidemics abroad. Africans in Dallas who spent time in the affected West African countries during the outbreak were thus witnesses of its negative consequences and of the challenges associated with disease control in the region. It was through their eyes that other Africans in Dallas experienced these events and were able to appreciate the seriousness of the crisis. On the one hand, therefore, transnational migrations will increase the risk of immigrants contracting viruses in other countries. On the other hand, it will provide migrants with experiences useful for increasing awareness of the scale of the problem while garnering support for action against viruses in their communities abroad.

Global migration movements could nevertheless continue to contribute to the spread of disease, even in the absence of such transnational connections. The intuition behind this perspective was one that made it easy for critics to invoke the influence of migration in their attempt to understand how an Ebola-infected patient traveling to the United States for the first time was diagnosed with the disease in Dallas. Ignoring the nuances of the relationship between these one-way migrations and disease makes it difficult to appreciate the complexity of the factors that made this possible. For example, migration from Liberia to the United States depends on a global infrastructure supporting international air travel, economic ties between countries, and improved technologies for conducting international communications. However, these same factors are part of the foundation on which international cooperation is built and influence much of the social dynamics observed in contemporary global communities. Accordingly, they make positive contributions to economic growth, support humanitarian operations, and facilitate the transportation of resources needed for combatting the spread of disease.

On balance, therefore, the contributions of these global processes far outweigh the potential risk they create for the transmission of disease. When these transmissions occur, societies will be faced with very little choice but to develop ways in which to respond. Because of the contributions of global migrations to the growth of immigrant communities, these responses are likely to include negative reactions toward these communities for the transmission of diseases perceived to be linked to their origin countries. Such responses have defined the majority of what was observed in prior epidemics tied to immigrants and were relevant to understanding the social response to the African immigrant community during the outbreak in Dallas.

Immigrants, Epidemics, and American Social Responses

In the past century, American communities have routinely demonstrated the salience of such responses during epidemics. They occurred against a backdrop of economic progress and robust increases in American living standards achieved during the Industrial Revolution. Owing to these increases in American prosperity, the country experienced one of the largest increases in immigration in its history. With an average of 4.5 million immigrants arriving per decade between 1880 and 1900, immigration flows were occurring at a rate that was more than eight times higher than that observed in the early 1800s (Fix and Passel 1994). New immigrant communities soon emerged in major urban industrial centers, including cities such as Boston, Detroit, and New York. Of this group, it was New York that became one of the most important locations where epidemics tied to these new immigrants were observed.

One of them occurred between May 8 and May 9, 1916, after two children were infected with polio in the city's Italian immigrant community (Wyatt 2011). Although the disease was present in the city before then, the diagnosis marked the beginning of a major polio epidemic that subsequently spread to other neighborhoods. Given the high incidence of the disease in the Italian immigrant community, the ensuing social crisis was defined by the blaming of Italians and the stigmatization of residents of their community (Wyatt 2011). Apparently, there were few systematic responses observed among immigrants in the community. Part of this was due to their extreme disadvantage, marked by their overcrowded neighborhoods and marginalization for practicing strange customs, such as the kissing of the dead (Kraut 2010).

Less than two decades prior, a similar set of events was observed on the West Coast of the United States. On March 6, 1900, the body of a Chinese laborer was found in the basement of a Chinatown hotel in San Francisco, and a subsequent examination of the corpse suggested that it had been infected with the plague bacilli (Risse 1992).* Like the death of the two Italian children infected with polio in 1916, this discovery was the physical event that was linked with the start of the epidemic in the city. However, the true origins of the epidemic were found abroad. Before then, the plague had been rapidly spreading in the Pacific region and other parts of Asia before it arrived in the United States through infected rats transported by ships (Markel 2009). The start of the epidemic in San Francisco created a social crisis that once again targeted the immigrant groups perceived to be linked to the physical event. Driven by the fear of the disease, a total quarantine was imposed on the city's Chinatown, while Chinese immigrants were extensively stigmatized (Risse 1992).

More than a century later, an identical sequence of events was observed in Dallas—within a context of widespread immigration, just as the epidemics of the early 1900s had been. This time, however, the immigrant groups were more diverse. Like these prior epidemics, the arrival of the Ebola virus in Dallas was also tied to the most widely used means of international travel of our time. When Duncan died at the THP hospital, his

---

* According to Trauner (1978), the autopsy revealed that the deceased had enlarged lymph nodes, and as a result, the plague was considered to be a probable cause of death.

death became the physical event that initiated the local crisis connected to immigrants from Africa. However, in absolute terms, the number of Ebola-infected persons in Dallas was smaller than the numbers of infected persons observed in either the polio or the plague epidemics. Nevertheless, the subsequent social crisis was no different. It was started by events that occurred in a well-known context of socioeconomic disadvantage (i.e., Vickery Meadow). It revolved around a fear of death that was made worse by misinformation about the channels through which the disease was transmitted. It also involved the blaming of Africans as well as the invoking of racist stereotypes to stigmatize them as people with infected bodies.

Significantly, however, the similarities between the Ebola crisis and epidemics observed in the early 1900s only extend so far because the social response to the events in Dallas had other unique features. For example, it was influenced by a unique social history of the racialization of African-origin populations in America. In contrast to Italian and Chinese immigrants in the 1900s, African immigrants belonged to a group that had been racialized as being inferior and stereotyped as having poor health for more than three centuries. At least in terms of perceptions, Ebola was also considered deadlier than diseases such as polio. Before the outbreak in Dallas, such perceptions had lingered in the American psyche as a result of fictional accounts of Ebola's relationship with horror, death, and mass destruction. The fear of Ebola was therefore around well before the arrival of Duncan but became more immediate after his death. Finally, the Ebola outbreak occurred in a context of real-time news reporting of the epidemic in West Africa and of the thousands of lives lost to the disease. Because of this, public awareness about the global consequences of the disease was increased in ways that were impossible to do in the early 1900s.

Thankfully, the outbreak in Dallas was eventually contained. However, there remains a fair chance that American communities will face the choice of how to respond to such events in the future. Technology will continue to improve, while the means of international travel will continue to change. Nevertheless, as long as countries remain connected by globalization and international migration continues to occur, the transmission of viruses between societies is likely to continue. The development of more effective strategies to control viral transmissions will be important for reducing the scale of these humanitarian crises. These strategies will remain important because emerging infectious diseases are challenging the limits of the global health apparatus. Unless their weak healthcare systems are improved, developing countries will remain some of the major sources from which these epidemics will emerge. This does not imply that more developed countries will not be the origins of such global epidemics; rather, it is an acknowledgment of the need to address the real problems that hamper the control of infectious diseases in resource-poor countries.

Disease outbreaks originating from countries abroad invariably create circumstances that increase public attention to immigrants from these countries. This trend will continue in the near future as long as the United States continues to be a major destination for immigrants. When these outbreaks occur, it will be important to understand what this attention will imply for the welfare of immigrant communities. A greater understanding of their consequences will also require a recognition that native-born populations could have a different set of responses to these events compared to immigrants themselves. Some of these responses would be adversarial, but others would not. This more comprehensive perspective is important and will form an objective basis for drawing conclusions about the social response to epidemics.

Revisiting the Dynamics of Social Responses to Epidemics

Alcabes's (2010) perspective on the unfolding of this response emphasizes the need to understand the physical event, the subsequent social crisis, and the narrative developed to understand the crisis. However, the evidence reviewed so far points to several ways that the response to the outbreak in Dallas was different than the response to previous epidemics. First, the social response was triggered by not one but two sets of physical events. The first was the *distal* event in West Africa, which African immigrants experienced by virtue of their transnational connections with the region. It was distal in the sense that it did not occur in their immediate locality. The second was the *proximate* physical event, defined by the death of Thomas Duncan in Dallas and the start of the outbreak in the city. As globalization increases, epidemics that stir social responses in immigrant communities will increasingly be characterized by outbreaks in two or more places. While this was partly true of many historical epidemics linked to immigrants, they did not occur in a context of globalization that was so advanced as to allow them to function as transnational actors with connections to diverse locations.

A second way in which the responses observed in Dallas differed was in terms of the narratives developed to understand the outbreak. Prior accounts of such narratives underscore the importance of blaming as a tool used by local natives to understand the causes of crises (Littleton et al. 2010; Nelkin and Gilman 1998). As shown throughout this book, this strategy was also employed by local natives responding to Africans in Dallas. This perspective is nevertheless limited by its focus on only one dimension of the development of these narratives. A second dimension of this response was the development of immigrants' own narrative of blame. Based on a different understanding of the causes of the crisis compared to those understood by the public, it focused on the influence of institutional arrangements such as the healthcare system and systems of racial discrimination. This multidimensional perspective indicates that narratives developed to help people understand that the causes of epidemics are more complex than is typically assumed. This complexity reflects the fact that the causes of epidemics can be interpreted quite differently by groups found within affected communities. As such, it is difficult to develop consensus around a specific set of factors perceived to be responsible for the spread of disease.

A third difference observed in Dallas is that the social response to the crisis did not just end with the process of blaming. Instead, it continued with an effort to push back against the social forces that threatened to afflict the African community. The most distinguishing feature of African immigrants' response, therefore, was their ability to develop counteractions. In taking these actions, they demonstrated their agency in making choices aimed at producing a positive change to the circumstances they confronted (Ruger 2004). Rather than allowing the backlash against them to push them into inaction, they became actively involved in tackling the consequences of the epidemic across various contexts.

By taking these actions, the African community in Dallas also showed that it was resilient. Contesting the forces that threatened their community required a resolve to fight back, and this they did. They pushed back against these forces despite the fact that they were otherized by locals, stigmatized as infected, and afflicted by the emotional toll of their concern for the affected countries. This resilience was fostered by decades of experience tackling a plethora of problems confronted by members of their community. They built effective institutions and cultivated systems of social support. Moreover, they exploited the benefits of bounded solidarity to address their common challenges. This is not to say that their resilience was solely driven by the resources found within their community. While these resources were important, they also appropriated other resources that they received from partnerships formed with institutions across the city.

Rarely has this ability of immigrants to challenge the status quo or mitigate the negative consequences of epidemics been acknowledged in previous studies. Indeed, we know very little about the actions of French immigrants in Germany or Italian immigrants in France after both groups were blamed for the spread of syphilis (Nelkin and Gilman 1988). Systematic accounts of the responses of Italian immigrants to combat the consequences of the polio epidemic are also largely unavailable, as are accounts of the agency shown by Chinese immigrants during the plague epidemic. This trend remains unchanged in recent studies of contemporary outbreaks linked to immigrants, including those associated with HIV/AIDS, SARS, and the Zika virus. In each case, coverage of the outbreak provides critical insight into the role of stereotypes, stigma, and blaming in shaping the perceptions of immigrants.* As such, it falls short of highlighting the ways that immigrants deal with these responses and bounce back from the ensuing social crisis.

What, then, explains these gaps in our understanding of immigrants' responses to the social consequences of epidemics? Why do we know so little about their efforts to recover from these events? The specific reasons for this are unclear, although possible answers can be found in a number of factors. For example, getting access to information on immigrant communities during epidemics is difficult, especially when they are at the center of the crisis created by the precipitating events. As a result of increased anti-immigrant sentiments, the threat to immigrants' lives can be so se-

---

* More discussion on the stigma, blame, and stereotypes associated with the SARS epidemic is provided by Eichelberger (2007) and Siu (2008). Similar discussions for Zika are provided by McNeil (2016) and for HIV/AIDS by Fairchild and Tynan (1994).

vere that it warrants a retreat from public displays of agency. Accordingly, Chinese immigrants in San Francisco would have had very little incentive to organize meaningful counteractions after living in quarantine and learning of threats to burn down their residences (Risse 2017). Another possibility is that the historical circumstances in which prior epidemics occurred imposed constraints to immigrants' interaction with their origin countries in ways that would have provided limited support for an international response. In the early 1900s, for example, transportation networks were comparatively underdeveloped, global travel more expensive, and the infrastructure to support transnationalism too weak to allow immigrants to participate in the social life of multiple countries. All told, the possible factors that explain the limited focus on immigrant agency during previous epidemics are diverse, and the specific ways that they undermined immigrant responses are undetermined. However, the end result of these gaps in knowledge is clear—the creation of a perception of inaction among immigrants and the implication that they are resigned to the influence of the negative forces directed toward their community.

Explaining the African Response in Dallas

Given this perception of inaction, it is important to understand why we observed clear patterns of prosocial action among African immigrants in Dallas. After all, they were targeted by similar acts of discrimination and had to confront many of the same negative reactions from the public as those experienced by immigrants in the early 1900s. What explains their ability to garner support in their fight against the epidemic in Africa? What were the central institutional arrangements in their community that supported the initiatives they took to address the disruption caused by the outbreak?

A useful place to start searching for answers is the examination of the differences in the social and demographic characteristics of recent African immigrants and those of immigrants in the epidemics of the early 1900s. Compared to the latter, African immigrants have much higher levels of human capital. Like many other recent immigrants, they are more educated and more highly skilled compared to the European groups that arrived at the turn of the twentieth century (Healey 2010). Notwithstanding their stratification into distinct groups of highly and poorly educated individuals, African immigrants collectively account for some of the highest levels of schooling in the United States (Capps et al. 2012). It was the members of the highly educated strata of these immigrants who provided much of the leadership used to develop responses that were observed in the community. These immigrants were businessmen, church leaders, entrepreneurs, and educators who had prior leadership experience in the city. Therefore, the African immigrant community had a cadre of professionals with the skills required to manage organizations, promote initiatives, and execute planned responses to the city's Ebola outbreak. Evidence on the presence of such a highly skilled group among the immigrant groups affected by the epidemics of the early 1900s is generally unavailable. Unlike Italians or Chinese immigrants, most African immigrants also arrive in the United States with high levels of English proficiency by virtue of their origins in English-speaking countries (Capps et al. 2012). Along with their language attributes and professional resources, they knew how to interact with media institutions, where to seek legal redress for acts of discrimination, and how to organize forums to reach out to the public during the outbreak in Dallas.

Because many of these immigrants were fairly well integrated into Dallas society, they were also embedded into social networks that provided them with access to other resources outside their community. As such, they could collaborate with mainstream churches and had relationships with humanitarian groups that contributed to the local and international campaign against the epidemic. By contrast, available descriptions of early European immigrant communities afflicted by epidemics suggest that most of them lacked access to these social connections. They were poor, lived in isolated communities, and largely lacked meaningful connections with institutions that could provide resources to help mitigate the health crisis in their communities.

Importantly, however, the mere availability of these resources in Dallas did not imply that African immigrants had access to them. In other words, without the goodwill of Americans who were sympathetic to their plight, the scale of their overall responses would have been limited. This goodwill illustrates key nuances in the ways in which local communities respond to immigrants blamed for the spread of disease. Put differently, local goodwill demonstrated that acts of benevolence could still be found in contexts of fear and widespread blaming of immigrants. These benevolent actions were important for providing complementary resources needed to ameliorate the circumstances of African immigrants. They included the provision of material support by local hospitals and the willingness of some locals to use payroll deductions to contribute to the international response initiated by the African community.

We cannot discount the contribution of transnationalism as an additional explanation for African immigrants' ability to respond more extensively to the consequences of the epidemic. Their dual connection to life in the United States and in Africa was more than just nominal commitments to participate in communities located on both sides of the Atlantic. It involved making investments, building institutions, and maintaining relationships with others in their origin countries. It involved cultivating connections between their origin countries and their community in Dallas to promote development in Africa. The infrastructure created to maintain these connections subsequently became useful for the accumulation and deployment of resources between Dallas and West Africa. This suggests that increased transnationalism among contemporary immigrants could foster the development of connections that could play a critical role in global crises in the future.

Finally, African immigrants had functional institutions that were developed in previous decades to address routine crises in their community and in Africa. Growing African settlement in the city and the barriers they encountered in their efforts to integrate had led to the development of such mechanisms to address the welfare of members of their community. Even though they were developed to provide specific functions, African immigrant institutions remained open to performing eclectic roles that allowed them to adapt to the changing needs of their community. When tragedies afflicted their members, they adapted to provide essential support to those in need. When faced with the global consequences of civil conflict in Africa, they adjusted to meet the needs of refugees arriving in the city. In fact, it was while providing these functions that they first started serving refugees from the three countries that were later at the center of the epidemic in West Africa. Both functionally and socially, therefore, African immigrant institutions provided a critical foundation for developing a response to the crisis. There was no need for the community to create new mechanisms for dealing with the epidemic. As a result, they simply built on the foundations laid by these institutions in ways that were crucial for demonstrating their resilience.

Theoretical Implications

Of the many implications that can be drawn from the analysis of the crisis in Dallas, the most important is the need for improved frameworks for understanding how immigrants respond to epidemics. The evidence presented so far suggests that this can be done in at least two ways. The first is to develop a broader understanding of the places *where* these responses are observed. Much of the previous attention given to these responses focuses on what occurs in immigrant destination countries. However, this approach is limited and inadequately recognizes the international dimensions of epidemics and the global interconnectedness of immigrants' social lives. Unlike immigrants in the past, who maintained comparatively weak ties with their origin countries, the ties maintained by recent immigrants are more enduring. As a result, social disruptions that affect the lives of contemporary immigrants during epidemics will be increasingly observed in communities found in both their origin and destination countries.

A second way to improve frameworks for understanding these social responses is to pay attention to question of *who* is responding. The difficulties of accessing information from immigrant communities should not be allowed to lead to an exclusive focus on the responses of native-born populations toward immigrants. One lesson we learn from the crisis in Dallas is that the significance of immigrants during these periods extends beyond their role in being the targets of blame and stigma. Whether it was through the development of their own narratives or in the steps they took to deal with stigma, the African immigrant community showed that immigrants can also be actively involved in responses observed at every stage of an epidemic. Another set of actors that will require more attention are nationals in the immigrant-origin countries where epidemics emerge. These actors are essential because they underscore the importance of transnational collaborations for the success of interventions initiated by immigrants abroad. As mentioned earlier, these collaborations are not necessarily new and are alluded to in studies on immigrant forays into social development in their origin countries. However, they are rarely examined during humanitarian emergencies or discussed in ways that illustrate their importance to the success of immigrants' philanthropic endeavors.

Beyond these conceptual issues, more comprehensive approaches are needed to understand the processes of blame and stigma. If the crisis in Dallas tells us anything, it is that these processes are more complicated than is typically assumed. On one level, they include traditional notions of blame and stigma as responses that co-occur during outbreaks of disease. As with leprosy, syphilis, and other infectious diseases, therefore, the stigma of Ebola was rooted in reactions defined by the fear of infection and subsequent death. On another level, the Ebola crisis showed that the stigmatized could also deploy other types of stigma themselves. Taken together, these observations suggest that the deployment of stigma occurs along multiple pathways that can originate among a diverse set of actors.

This diversity does not imply that the implications of stigma are the same regardless of the source of its deployment. It still remains true that stigmas have more negative consequences when deployed by more powerful groups to ostracize the less powerful. For instance, African immigrants faced social disadvantages associated with their status as immigrants and their status as racial minorities before being used as targets of stigma. As a result, the consequences of these stigmas accentuated their disadvantaged status in ways that had negative effects on the lives of Africans in other US states. Compared to these consequences, the effects of stigma deployed within the African community were relatively minor. They involved trivial differences in social status, were observed less frequently, and were generally less consequential.

Another theoretical implication of the analysis is the continued significance of racial and ethnic disadvantage demonstrated in this book. It was seen in the use of racial and ethnic markers to identify targets of stigma. It was observed in the ways in which racist views about Black health were so easily invoked to otherize African immigrants as carriers of disease. This evidence indicates that historical stereotypes of Blackness and their relationship with disease still remain a fundamental part of American understanding of the health outcomes of African-origin populations. In this case, stereotypes about the inferior health of Black slaves were replaced with cultural caricatures used to dehumanize African immigrants over the course of the epidemic.

That these factors remain relevant for understanding the social experiences of African immigrants confirms the predictions of immigration theorists who emphasize the significance of racial and ethnic disadvantage for the incorporation of Black immigrants. In contrast to classical assimilation theorists who focus on the experiences of early European immigrants, these theorists predict, among other things, that racial and ethnic minority status will create a significant barrier to the social integration of more recent immigrant groups (Portes and Zhou 1993). The ease with which narratives of racial inferiority were invoked to develop a narrative of poor African immigrant health showed that this barrier remains a central part of Black immigrants' experiences. Additionally, the crisis in the city only showed how the effect of this influence was heightened during the epidemic. Before this period, experiences of racism and prejudice were a central part of African immigrants' daily experiences, and this is unlikely to change after their recovery from the crisis.

Equally important is the need to pay more attention to the questions of resistance and contestation in research on immigrant health. Socially marginalized groups do not always succumb to the status quo nor do they always yield to institutionalized structures of inequality. Previous studies thus document the activities of resistance movements and the political struggles of marginalized populations associated with the fight against colonialism (Featherstone 2013; Frost and Hoggett 2008; Prakash et al. 1994). Despite the abundance of this evidence, however, it is surprising that the analysis of such actions has received limited attention in accounts of epidemics. African immigrants' responses illustrate two features of these actions that are important for health research. The first is that acts of resistance, such as the use of deception, are not always visible to members of the groups being resisted. The second is that immigrant communities possess diverse resources that can be used to organize responses to challenge the negative forces that threaten their existence.

Implications for Policy

Identifying policy implications of the experiences of the African immigrant community is complicated, in part, because the circumstances in which they occurred are not representative of all cases of disease outbreaks among immigrants. Despite this limitation, we can glean a number of insights from these events, which can provide the building blocks for the development of appropriate interventions. One such insight relates to the usefulness of the responses of these immigrants for emphasizing the importance of community-led efforts of disease control. Usually, the main strategies used to combat disease transmission during epidemics draw heavily from the work of international health bureaucracies. Led by institutions such as the WHO, these institutions manage and control the global spread of disease based on the advice of experts and their years of experience working to improve global health. While this approach has been successful in many cases (e.g., WHOWG 2006), it is not always the most appropriate for fostering grassroots involvement in disease control. One reason for this is that it focuses on top-down strategies of disease control rather than on incorporating the advantages of bottom-up initiatives. Global efforts of disease control can thus be improved by giving greater recognition to the knowledge systems, resources, and institutions found within local communities. This recognition is important for improving the capacity of these communities to provide a first line of defense against the spread of disease.

As we learned from the outbreak in Dallas, immigrant communities are both willing and able to act to provide such grassroots-level interventions. Rather than wait for help from public health bureaucracies, the African community started thinking about how to stop the spread of Ebola in the very early stages of the epidemic. It began with an effort to lobby government officials in Africa to act more decisively to control the spread of the virus. After the start of the local outbreak, it continued with their decision to take action to prevent the spread of infection, promote good health practices, and educate others about Ebola. These actions suggest that residents of local communities have the potential to become rudimentary health workers who could be used in the fight against infectious diseases (Delacollette et al. 1996; Maes and Kalofonos 2013). However, this potential cannot be realized without the engagement of these communities and a commitment to view them as partners and not as sources of fear. It will also require a willingness to collaborate with them and identify the resources they possess, which can be used to increase their capacity to respond during health crises.

Finding innovative methods to develop the potential of immigrant institutions is one way that these objectives can be achieved. The African immigrant response illustrated the diversity of the roles these institutions play and the vast resources they possess for addressing larger goals of so- cial policy. Of particular importance is their ability to engage in collective action. Although specific types of action taken by these institutions have been observed in immigrant communities (e.g., Chen 2002; Takougang and Tidjani 2009; Zhou and Li 2003), the scale of the emergency created by the Ebola crisis warranted a mobilization of the resources of many immigrant organizations to address a common problem. Such demonstrations of collective action can be harnessed to tackle other important problems, including humanitarian disasters, homelessness, and the social consequences of crime. Furthermore, the ability of African immigrant organizations to collaborate with mainstream institutions highlights other ways that the potential of these organizations can be developed: for example, the cultivation of partnerships between these organizations and outside groups, their integration into local systems of social service provisioning, and the expansion of their potential to reach underserved populations.

Unfortunately, in accordance with the dynamics of issue-attention cycles (Peters and Hogwood 1985; Petersen 2009), public attention shifted away from the African immigrant community after the end of the Ebola epidemic. This shift was accompanied by a decline in the participation of local institutions in humanitarian activity in Africa. Given the high likelihood that other epidemics will occur among immigrants in the future, more should be done to prepare immigrant institutions to respond to these events. Continued transnational migration between the United States and the developing world suggests, for example, that immigrant institutions can play an important role in the provision of disease surveillance among sick immigrants returning from visits abroad.

To achieve this objective, it will be important to invest in leadership development to further strengthen the capacity of these institutions. It is concerning that much of the leadership of the ethnic institutions that led the response to the Dallas outbreak was provided by professionals and other socially mobile individuals. Few marginalized groups have a substantial cadre of such professionals, and as a result, the replication of these efforts in the future is likely to be challenging. Unlike African immigrants, for example, many immigrants from Latin America and the Caribbean have low levels of education, as well as some of the lowest levels of occupational attainment in the United States (Zong and Batalova 2016). Other groups, such as immigrants from Iraq and Afghanistan, are similarly disadvantaged in terms of their low levels of English proficiency and employment, and their relative social isolation (GAO 2018). In addition, they lack the benefit of living in communities with conationals who are highly skilled professionals with connections outside their communities. In the absence of interventions to improve their socioeconomic circumstances, their ability to respond to future epidemics will be limited. However, these limits can be overcome by building the capacity of immigrant institutions and preparing to better serve their communities.

None of this should distract us from the need for stronger interventions to contain epidemics abroad. Opportunities to preempt the Dallas crisis were missed, in part, because of the poor management of the initial response in West Africa. Not only was the response to the Ebola outbreak in Meliandou inadequate, but the absence of disease surveillance teams on the borders of Guinea made it easy for infected persons to travel to neighboring countries. In each of the affected countries, the spread of Ebola was further affected by weak healthcare systems, which were unable to contain the spread of the disease, and this culminated in the failure to diagnose Duncan as a possibly infected patient before he boarded his flight for the United States. Many of these systemic failures are now recognized in existing studies (Boozary et al. 2014; Gates 2015; Gostin and Friedman 2015). What remains is the need for more focused investments in the healthcare systems of developing countries, especially those in Africa, and the improvement of measures to identify travelers infected with a disease before their departure. Complementary investments are also needed in American border institutions to help them be better prepared to identify infected persons at various ports of entry. Together with their counterparts in other countries, these institutions can provide another line of defense to mitigate the spread of infections that could be transmitted by travelers.

At the same time, the African immigrant response in Dallas further showed us why it is important for immigrant-origin countries to develop strategies to harness diaspora resources during periods of humanitarian emergency. The foundation of these strategies exists in the form of national efforts to encourage diaspora groups to participate in development efforts in their homelands. However, these efforts could be complemented with two additional strategies. The first is to be very deliberate in narrowing the scope of these efforts during periods of national crisis. Rather than simply seeking resources from diaspora groups to improve their economies, the governments of developing countries should use these periods to request specific types of resources that can be used to respond to these crises. The second is to advance mechanisms for improving the dual flow of information between immigrants and their origin-country governments. As shown in the experiences of Africans in Dallas, diaspora interventions are more enhanced when they are linked with information received on critical needs in origin home countries that could be better addressed with resources from abroad.

Opportunities for Future Research

Global connections between societies will ensure that the relationship among migration, health, and disease continues to remain a central part of studies on the social implications of epidemics. While this book presents an account of the relevance of this relationship among contemporary African immigrants, the relationship observed in future studies will most likely be shaped by a different set of realities. Still, the account presented in this book can be used to identify several issues that could be addressed in future studies. One of these is the question of how the responses observed in local communities are influenced by the scale of disease epidemics. Given that Duncan was the only person, indeed the only African, who died from Ebola in Dallas, it is important to address the hypothetical question of what types of community responses will be observed in contexts with more fatalities. For now, the extent to which immigrants are willing to develop prosocial responses to outbreaks with such fatalities remains unclear. Mounting fatalities could intensify community reactions of prejudice against immigrants in ways that could significantly undermine their ability to show displays of agency. Therefore, insights from future studies will improve our understanding of immigrant responses to mass casualty events, the limits of agency during quarantines, and the dynamics of immigrant-native partnerships under extreme disease conditions.

Immigration research could benefit from the expansion of studies that examine the centrality of immigrant institutions to life in immigrant communities. In light of the eclectic nature of the functions provided by African immigrant institutions, more research is needed to examine the range of nontraditional functions provided by these institutions that help to buffer their communities during periods of crisis. Perhaps these functions could be leveraged to address the plight of children migrating as unaccompanied minors or the welfare of victims of trafficking. However, these potentials cannot be realized without a better understanding of how these institutions operate. Future studies also need to provide insight into the determinants of the effectiveness of these institutions during periods of adversity. This will require new studies on the significance of their leadership styles, patterns of membership, and transnational connections in shaping their ability to act under conditions of duress.

Additionally, more diverse global contexts need to be incorporated into research on how immigrants respond to epidemics. Despite the challenges they experience during their incorporation into society, immigrants in the United States can arguably tap into comparatively more community resources to mobilize such responses than immigrants in the developing world. In many poor countries, immigrants have lower levels of human capital, earn comparatively lower incomes, and do not have the same opportunities for social mobility as immigrants in the United States. Indeed, their comparative disadvantage is seen in studies showing that the size of migrant remittances sent from the United States far exceeds that sent by immigrants in developing countries (World Bank 2017).* Developing-country contexts are also important for understanding specific nuances in the relationship between migration and disease. For example, cross-border migrations between Guinea, Liberia, and Sierra Leone occurred as part of long-standing traditions of international migration. As a result, they raise important questions concerning the role of transnationalism in immigrant responses to epidemics in such contexts.

Within the United States, future epidemics are likely to provide new opportunities to investigate whether the responses of Africans in Dallas are similar to those that will be initiated by other contemporary immigrant groups. Such studies will strengthen the foundations for reversing the per-

* This information was found via the World Bank's World Development Indicators database (https://datacatalog.worldbank.org/dataset/world-development-indicators).

ception of immigrants as relatively passive observers to crises that negatively affect their communities. No longer should the focus of research on these epidemics revolve around themes of immigrant victimhood and indifference. Depending on the availability of reliable data, future studies could even reevaluate what we know about historical epidemics to assess the evidence on immigrant agency in the face of stigma. Perhaps these historical studies discounted evidence on immigrant agency to instead focus on the challenges that emerge when immigrants are the public face of epidemics. Perhaps the scope of action available to these immigrants was truly constrained by the social and historical circumstances in which they occurred. What the response of Africans in Dallas tells us is that these circumstances may no longer restrict the options for action available to immigrants in the United States. Rather than being passive victims, they are proactive participants who take decisive action to counter the social forces that disrupt life in their communities.

References

Abeysinghe, Sudeepa. 2016. "Ebola at the borders: Newspaper representations and the politics of border control." *Third World Quarterly* 37, no. 3: 452–467.

Abramowitz, Sharon Alane, Kristen E. McLean, Sarah Lindley McKune, Kevin Louis Bardosh, Mosoka Fallah, Josephine Monger, Kodjo Tehoungue, and Patricia A. Omidian. 2015. "Community-centered responses to Ebola in urban Liberia: The view from below." *PLoS Neglected Tropical Diseases* 9, no. 4: e0003706.

Adeyanju, Charles T., and Nicole Neverson. 2007. "'There will be a next time': Media discourse about an 'apocalyptic' vision of immigration, racial diversity, and health risks." *Canadian Ethnic Studies* 39, nos. 1–2: 79–105.

Adeyanju, Charles T., and Temitope Oriola. 2010. "Not in Canada: The non-Ebola panic and media misrepresentation of the Black community." *African Journal of Criminology and Justice Studies* 4, no. 1: 32–54.

Adger, W. Neil, Terry P. Hughes, Carl Folke, Stephen R. Carpenter, and Johan Rockström. 2005. "Social-ecological resilience to coastal disasters." *Science* 309, no. 5737: 1036–1039.

Aguilera, Michael B., and Douglas S. Massey. 2003. "Social capital and the wages of Mexican migrants: New hypotheses and tests." *Social Forces* 82, no. 2: 671–701.

Alba, Richard, and Victor Nee. 1997. "Rethinking assimilation theory for a new era of immigration." *International Migration Review* 34, no. 4: 826–874.

Alcabes, Philip. 2009. *Dread: How fear and fantasy have fueled epidemics from the Black Death to avian flu.* New York: Public Affairs.

Ali, Ihotu. 2011. "Staying off the bottom of the melting pot: Somali refugees respond to a changing US immigration climate." *Bildhaan: An International Journal of Somali Studies* 9, no. 1: 82–114.

Al-Jabban, Jihad. 2014. "Ebola: The political tool of biological agents." *Huffington Post*, November 18. http://www.huffingtonpost.com/jihad-aljabban/ebola-the-political-tool-_b_6175638.html.

Almendrala, Anna. 2015. "If Ebola hits again, this state is doing everything right."

Huffington Post, September 11. http://www.huffingtonpost.com/entry/ebola
-preparedness-state-minnesota_us_55e73f64e4b0c818f61a3a00.

Anderson, Mark. 2014. "Ebola: Airlines cancel more flights to affected countries."
The Guardian, August 22. https://www.theguardian.com/society/2014/aug/22
/ebola-airlines-cancel-flights-guinea-liberia-sierra-leone.

Arnold, David. 1991. "The Indian Ocean as a disease zone, 1500–1950." *South
Asia: Journal of South Asian Studies* 14, no. 2: 1–21.

Ayala, Eva-Marie, and Naheed Rajwani. 2014. "Dallas nurse receives transfusion
from Ebola survivor Dr. Kent Brantly." *Dallas News*, October 12. https://www
.dallasnews.com/news/news/2014/10/12/dallas-nurse-receives-transfusion
-from-ebola-survivor-dr.-kent-brantly.

Baba, Hana. 2014. "Bay Area Africans feel, and fight, Ebola stigma." *KALW Local
Public Radio*, December 16. http://kalw.org/post/bay-area-africans-feel-and
-fight-ebola-stigma#stream/0.

Baffoe, Michael, and Lewis Asimeng-Boahene. 2013. "Using cultural artifacts,
positions, and titles as retentions of cultural attachments to original homelands: African immigrants in the diaspora." *Academic Journal of Interdisci-
plinary Studies* 2, no. 2: 85–92.

Bah, Par, and Zoom Dosso. 2014. "Medics vent anger at government inaction
over Ebola." *Yahoo News*, June 26. https://www.yahoo.com/news/medics-vent
-anger-government-inaction-over-ebola-193234163.html?ref=gs.

Baize, Sylvain, Delphine Pannetier, Lisa Oestereich, Toni Rieger, Lamine
Koivogui, N'Faly Magassouba, Barrè Soropogui et al. 2014. "Emergence of
Zaire Ebola virus disease in Guinea." *New England Journal of Medicine* 371,
no. 15: 1418–1425.

Bakewell, Oliver, Hein De Haas, and Agnieszka Kubal. 2012. "Migration systems,
pioneer migrants and the role of agency." *Journal of Critical Realism* 11, no. 4:
413–437.

Balluck, Kyle. 2014. "ER nurse: Duncan lied about exposure to Ebola." *The Hill*,
October 26. http://thehill.com/policy/healthcare/221905-er-nurse-duncan
-lied-about-exposure-to-ebola.

Bandura, Albert. 2004. "Health promotion by social cognitive means." *Health
Education and Behavior* 31, no. 2: 143–164.

Bangura, John. 2016. "Hope in the midst of death: Charismatic spirituality,
healing evangelists, and the Ebola crisis in Sierra Leone." *Missionalia* 44,
no. 1: http://missionalia.journals.ac.za/pub/article/view/113/pdf.

Barde, Robert. 2004. "Plague in San Francisco: An essay review." *Journal of the
History of Medicine and Allied Sciences* 59, no. 3: 463–470.

Barquet, Nicolau, and Pere Domingo. 1997. "Smallpox: The triumph over the
most terrible of the ministers of death." *Annals of Internal Medicine* 127, no. 8:
635–642.

Belvedere, Matthew J. 2014. "How Ebola can quickly mutate: 'Hot Zone' author." *CNBC*, October 20. https://www.cnbc.com/2014/10/20/how-ebola-can -quickly-mutate-hot-zone-author.html.

Bennett, Brian. 2014. "US tightens travel restrictions from West Africa to curb Ebola." *Los Angeles Times*, October 21. http://www.latimes.com/nation/la-na -ebola-air-20141022-story.html.

Berman, Russell. 2014. "Democrats vs. Obama on an Ebola travel ban." *The Atlantic*, October 21. https://www.theatlantic.com/politics/archive/2014/10 /democrats-defy-obama-in-favor-of-ebola-travel-ban/381712/.

Bernstein, Sharon. 2014. "With Ebola fear running high, African immigrants face ostracism." *Reuters*, October 24. http://www.reuters.com/article/us -health-ebola-usa-xenophobia-idUSKCN0ID1J420141024.

Beukes, Susan. 2014. "Finding Ebola's 'patient zero.'" *The Guardian*, October 28. https://www.theguardian.com/world/2014/oct/28/ebola-virus-guinea-first -victim-patient-zero.

Bigo, Didier. 2002. "Security and immigration: Toward a critique of the govern- mentality of unease." *Alternatives* 27, no. 1: 63–92.

Bird, Sheryl Thorburn, and Laura M. Bogart. 2001. "Perceived race-based and socioeconomic status (SES)–based discrimination in interactions with health care providers." *Ethnicity and Disease* 11, no. 3: 554–563.

Blake, Matthew, and Wills Robinson. 2014. "'I have this Ebola stigma and no one will take me in': Thomas Eric Duncan's fiancée is left homeless and shunned more than a week after being cleared of the deadly virus." *Daily Mail*, October 31. http://www.dailymail.co.uk/news/article-2815645/I-Ebola-stigma-no-one -Ebola-victim-s-fianc-e-homeless-shunned-week-cleared-deadly-virus.html.

Blendon, Robert J., C. M. DesRoches, J. M. Benson, M. J. Herrmann, E. Mackie, and K. J. Weldon. 2003. "Project on biological security and the public, Har- vard School of Public Health: SARS survey." Boston: Harvard School of Public Health. https://cdn1.sph.harvard.edu/wp-content/uploads/sites/94 /2012/09/WP10SARSUS2.pdf.

Blustein, Jan, and Linda J. Weiss. 1998. "Visits to specialists under Medicare: Socioeconomic advantage and access to care." *Journal of Health Care for the Poor and Underserved* 9, no. 2: 153–169.

Body-Gendrot, Sophie. 2012. *Globalization, fear and insecurity: The challenges for cities north and south.* New York: Springer.

Boerma, Lindsey. 2014. "Republican congressman: Immigrant children might carry Ebola." *CBS News*, August 5. http://www.cbsnews.com/news/republican -congressman-immigrant-children-might-carry-ebola/.

Bonanno, George A., Samuel M. Y. Ho, Jane C. K. Chan, Rosalie S. Y. Kwong, Celia K. Y. Cheung, Claudia P. Y. Wong, and Vivian C. W. Wong. 2008. "Psychological resilience and dysfunction among hospitalized survivors of the SARS epidemic in Hong Kong: A latent class approach." *Health Psychology* 27, no. 5: 659.

Bonsu, Samuel K. 2009. "Colonial images in global times: Consumer interpretations of Africa and Africans in advertising." *Consumption, Markets and Culture* 12, no. 1: 1–25.

Bonsu, Samuel K., and Russell W. Belk. 2003. "Do not go cheaply into that good night: Death-ritual consumption in Asante, Ghana." *Journal of Consumer Research* 30, no. 1: 41–55.

Boozary, Andrew S., Paul E. Farmer, and Ashish K. Jha. 2014. "The Ebola outbreak, fragile health systems, and quality as a cure." *Jama* 312, no. 18: 1859–1860.

Brandt, Allan M. 1988. "The syphilis epidemic and its relation to AIDS." *Science* 239, no. 4838: 375–380.

Brantly, Kent, Amber Brantly, and David Thomas. 2015. *Called for life: How loving our neighbor led us to the heart of the Ebola epidemic.* Colorado Springs: Waterbrook Press.

Bravo, Vanessa. 2017. "Coping with dying and deaths at home: How undocumented migrants in the United States experience the process of transnational grieving." *Mortality* 22, no. 1: 33–44.

Brettell, Caroline B. 2005. "The spatial, social, and political incorporation of Asian Indian immigrants in Dallas, Texas." *Urban Anthropology and Studies of Cultural Systems and World Economic Development* 34, no. 2/3: 247–280.

Brettell, Caroline B. 2011. "Experiencing everyday discrimination: A comparison across five immigrant populations." *Race and Social Problems* 3, no. 4: 266–279.

Brettell, Caroline B., and Faith G. Nibbs. 2010. "Immigrant suburban settlement and the 'threat' to middle class status and identity: The case of Farmers Branch, Texas." *International Migration* 49, no. 1: 1–30.

Broderick, Cyril. 2014. "Ebola, AIDS manufactured by Western Pharmaceuticals, US DoD?" *Daily Observer*, September 9. https://www.liberianobserver.com /news/security/ebola-aids-manufactured-by-western-pharmaceuticals-us-dod/.

Brodsky, Betty. 1988. "Mental health attitudes and practices of Soviet Jewish immigrants." *Health and Social Work* 13, no. 2: 130–136.

Brown, DeNeen, and Pamela Constable. 2014. "West Africans in Washington say they are stigmatized because of Ebola fear." *Washington Post.* October 16. https://www.washingtonpost.com/local/west-africans-in-washington-say -they-are-being-stigmatized-because-of-ebola-fear/2014/10/16/39442d18 -54c6-11e4-892e-602188e70e9c_story.html.

Brown, Katrina, and Elizabeth Westaway. 2011. "Agency, capacity, and resilience to environmental change: Lessons from human development, well-being, and disasters." *Annual Review of Environment and Resources* 36 (2011): 321–342.

Butty, James. 2014. "Liberia announces additional Ebola containment measures." *Voice of America*, July 31. http://www.voanews.com/a/liberia-announces -additional-ebola-containment-measures/1968611.html.

Byrne, Matt. 2014. "Maine school board puts teacher on leave after she travelled to Dallas." *Press Herald*, October 17. http://www.pressherald.com/2014/10/17 /fearing-ebola-strong-elementary-teacher-on-leave-after-traveling-to-dallas/.

Capps, Randy, Kristen McCabe, and Michael Fix. 2012. "Diverse streams: African migration to the United States." Migration Policy Institute: Washington, DC. https://www.fcd-us.org/diverse-streams-african-migration-to-the-united -states/.

Casey, Logan. 2015. "Emotions and politics of Ebola." *Political Science and Politics* 48, no. 1: 7–8.

Cassidy, John. 2014. "The nightmarish politics of Ebola." *New Yorker*, October 9. http://www.newyorker.com/news/john-cassidy/politics-ebola-containment.

Castles, Stephen. 2004. "The factors that make and unmake migration policies 1." *International Migration Review* 38, no. 3: 852–884.

———. 2010. "Understanding global migration: A social transformation perspective." *Journal of Ethnic and Migration Studies* 36, no. 10: 1565–1586.

CBS News. 2014. "Ebola fear causes stigma against West Africans in U.S." *CBS News*, October 31. http://www.cbsnews.com/news/ebola-fear-causes-stigma -against-west-africans-in-u-s/.

Centers for Disease Control and Prevention (CDC). 1982. "Opportunistic infections and Kaposi's sarcoma among Haitians in the United States." *Morbidity and Mortality Weekly Report* 31, no. 26: 353–354.

———. 2003. "Update: Outbreak of severe acute respiratory syndrome worldwide, 2003." *Morbidity and Mortality Weekly Report* 52, no. 12: 241–246.

———. 2014. "Enhanced Ebola screening to start at five U.S. airports and new tracking program for all people entering U.S. from Ebola-affected countries." October 8. https://www.cdc.gov/media/releases/2014/p1008-ebola-screening .html.

Chan, Ivy W. S., Julian C. L. Lai, and Kris W. N. Wong. 2006. "Resilience is associated with better recovery in Chinese people diagnosed with coronary heart disease." *Psychology and Health* 21, no. 3: 335–349.

Chan, Kenneth. 2004. "African immigrant churches creating oases of faith." *Christian Post*, May 1. http://www.christianpost.com/news/african-immigrant -churches-creating-oases-of-faith-14906/.

Chang, David. 2014. "African students scheduled to start at NJ school will stay home past waiting period amid Ebola concerns." *NBC Philadelphia*. October 19. https://www.nbcphiladelphia.com/news/local/Ebola-Fears-and-Arrival -of-2-African-Students-Prompt-Parents-to-Keep-Kids-Home-From-Local -School--279718882.html.

Chen, Carolyn. 2002. "The religious varieties of ethnic presence: A comparison between a Taiwanese immigrant Buddhist temple and an evangelical Christian church." *Sociology of Religion* 63, no. 2: 215–238.

Chin, John J., Torsten B. Neilands, Linda Weiss, and Joanne E. Mantell. 2008. "Paradigm shifters, professionals, and community sentinels: Immigrant community institutions' roles in shaping places and implications for stigmatized public health initiatives." *Health and Place* 14, no. 4: 866–882.

Chishti, Muzaffar, Faye Hipsman, and Sarah Pierce. 2014. "Ebola outbreak rekindles debate on restricting admissions to the United States on health grounds." *Migration Policy Institute*, October 23. http://www.migrationpolicy.org/article/ebola-outbreak-rekindles-debate-restricting-admissions-united-states-health-grounds.

Cohen, Emma. 2015. "The 2014 Ebola epidemic and racial 'othering.'" *Georgetown University Journal of Health Sciences* 9: 4–14.

Cole, Teju. 2014. "What it is." *New Yorker*, October 7. http://www.newyorker.com/books/page-turner/what-is-ebola.

Cordell, Dennis D., and Manuel Garcia y Griego. 2005. "The integration of Nigerian and Mexican immigrants in Dallas/Fort Worth, Texas." Unpublished working paper. Princeton University. http://citeseerx.ist.psu.edu/viewdoc/download?doi=10.1.1.693.498&rep=rep1&type=pdf.

Cotler, S. J., S. Cotler, H. Xie, B. J. Luc, T. J. Layden, and S. S. Wong. 2012. "Characterizing hepatitis B stigma in Chinese immigrants." *Journal of Viral Hepatitis* 19, no. 2: 147–152.

Covey, Herbert C. 2001. "People with leprosy (Hansen's disease) during the Middle Ages." *Social Science Journal* 38, no. 2: 315–321.

Crocker, Jennifer, Brenda Major, and C. Steel. 1998. "Social stigma." In *The Handbook of Social Psychology*, 4th ed., edited by Daniel T. Gilbert, Susan T. Fiske, and Gardner Lindzey, 504–553. Oxford: Oxford University Press.

Cunha, B. A. 2002. "Anthrax, tularemia, plague, Ebola or smallpox as agents of bioterrorism: Recognition in the emergency room." *Clinical Microbiology and Infection* 8, no. 8: 489–503.

Cunningham, Solveig Argeseanu, Julia D. Ruben, and K. M. Venkat Narayan. 2008. "Health of foreign-born people in the United States: A review." *Health and Place* 14, no. 4: 623–635.

Curran, James W., and Harold W. Jaffe. 2011. "AIDS: The early years and CDC's response." *Morbidity and Mortality Weekly Report* 60, no. 4: 64–69.

Dai, Jia, and Kideuk Hyun. 2010. "Global risk, domestic framing: Coverage of the North Korean nuclear test by US, Chinese, and South Korean news agencies." *Asian Journal of Communication* 20, no. 3: 299–317.

Dallas Morning News. 2000. "Our Town: Vickery Meadow struggles with population explosion." November 19. 2J.

Dallas News Administrator. 2014. "Ebola briefs: City of Dallas releases audio of 911 call about Duncan." *Dallas News*, October. https://www.dallasnews.com /news/news/2014/10/14/ebola-briefs-city-of-dallas-releases-audio-of-911-call -about-duncan.

Darboe, K. 2003. "New immigrants in Minnesota: The Somali immigration and assimilation." *Journal of Developing Societies* 19, no. 4: 458–472.

Davis, Mark, Niamh Stephenson, and Paul Flowers. 2011. "Compliant, complacent or panicked? Investigating the problematisation of the Australian general public in pandemic influenza control." *Social Science and Medicine* 72, no. 6: 912–918.

Davis, Rebecca. 2014. "Ebola epidemic 2014: Timeline." *Guardian Africa Network*, October 15. https://www.theguardian.com/world/2014/oct/15/ebola -epidemic-2014-timeline.

Deacon, H., I. Stephney, and S. Prosalendis. 2005. *Understanding HIV/AIDS stigma: A theoretical and methodological analysis.* Cape Town: Human Sciences Research Council Press.

De Haas, Hein. 2010. "Migration and development: A theoretical perspective 1." *International Migration Review* 44, no. 1: 227–264.

Delacollette, Charles, Patrick Van Der Stuyft, and K. Molima. 1996. "Using community health workers for malaria control: Experience in Zaire." *Bulletin of the World Health Organization* 74, no. 4: 423–440.

Delaney, Arthur. 2014. "Justice Department warns against Ebola discrimination." *Huffington Post*, December 15. http://www.huffingtonpost.com/2014/12/15 /ebola-justice-department_n_6329660.html.

Dellplain, Laura. 2012. "Yellow, in peril: How public health discourse on tuberculosis (TB) reveals, refines, and reinforces the racial stigmatization of Asian Americans." PhD diss., Oberlin College.

Delumeau, Jean. 1990. *Sin and fear: The emergence of a Western guilt culture 13th-18th centuries.* New York: St. Martin's Press.

Dennis, Brady, and Peyton Craighill. 2014. "Ebola poll: Two-thirds of Americans worried about possible widespread epidemic in the U.S." *Washington Post*, October 14. https://www.washingtonpost.com/national/health-science/ebola -poll-two-thirds-of-americans-worried-about-possible-widespread-epidemic -in-us/2014/10/13/d0afd0ee-52ff-11e4-809b-8cc0a295c773_story.html?no redirect=on&utm_term=.772d8c8c8250.

De Roo, Ann, Bwaka Ado, Berthe Rose, Yves Guimard, Karolien Fonck, and Robert Colebunders. 1998. "Survey among survivors of the 1995 Ebola epidemic in Kikwit, Democratic Republic of Congo: Their feelings and experiences." *Tropical Medicine and International Health* 3, no. 11: 883–885.

Derose, Kathryn Pitkin, José J. Escarce, and Nicole Lurie. 2007. "Immigrants and health care: Sources of vulnerability." *Health Affairs* 26, no. 5: 1258–1268.

DeShaw, Pamela J. 2006. "Use of the emergency department by Somali immigrants and refugees." *Minnesota Medicine* 89, no. 8: 42–45.

Devine, Patricia G., E. Ashby Plant, and Kristen Harrison. 1999. "The problem of 'us' versus 'them' and AIDS stigma." *American Behavioral Scientist* 42, no. 7: 1212–1228.

DeWitte, S. N., M. H. Kurth, C. R. Allen, and I. Linkov. 2016. "Disease epidemics: Lessons for resilience in an increasingly connected world." *Journal of Public Health* 39, no. 2: 254–257.

Dionne, K. Y., and L. Seay. 2015. "Perceptions about Ebola in America: Othering and the role of knowledge about Africa." *Political Science and Politics* 48, no. 1: 6–7.

Dixon, Robyn. 2014. "Texas Ebola patient aided Liberian woman thought to have malaria." *Los Angeles Times*, October 2. http://www.latimes.com/world/africa/la-fg-ebola-liberia-20141003-story.html.

Dodoo, F. Nii-Amoo. 1997. "Assimilation differences among Africans in America." *Social Forces* 76, no. 2: 527–546.

Duhaime-Ross, Arielle. 2014. "Ebola panic is getting pretty racist." *The Verge*, October 8. https://www.theverge.com/2014/10/8/6941749/ebola-panic-is-getting-pretty-racist.

Dunham, Will. 2014. "U.S. lawmakers blast government's Ebola response, urge travel ban." *Reuters*, October 16. http://www.reuters.com/article/us-health-ebola-usa-idUSKCN0I517E20141016.

Dysart-Gale, Deborah. 2007. "Clinicians and medical interpreters: Negotiating culturally appropriate care for patients with limited English ability." *Family and Community Health* 30, no. 3: 237–246.

Eichelberger, Laura. 2007. "SARS and New York's Chinatown: The politics of risk and blame during an epidemic of fear." *Social Science and Medicine* 65, no. 6: 1284–1295.

Elder Jr., Glen H. 1994. "Time, human agency, and social change: Perspectives on the life course." *Social Psychology Quarterly* 57, no. 1: 4–15.

Elgot, Jessica. 2014. "Nancy Writebol, the nurse who survived Ebola, reveals many are still too afraid to shake her hand." *Huffington Post UK*, November 24. http://www.huffingtonpost.co.uk/2014/11/24/ebola-nurse-nancy-writebol_n_6211758.html.

Ellis, B. Heidi, Helen Z. MacDonald, Alisa K. Lincoln, and Howard J. Cabral. 2008. "Mental health of Somali adolescent refugees: The role of trauma, stress, and perceived discrimination." *Journal of Consulting and Clinical Psychology* 76, no. 2: 184–193.

Ellison, Charles E. 2014. "Where Ebola meets concerns over race, class, and the uninsured." *The Root*, October 6. http://www.theroot.com/where-ebola-meets-concerns-over-race-class-and-the-uni-1790877283.

Emirbayer, Mustafa, and Ann Mische. 1998. "What is agency?" *American Journal of Sociology* 103, no. 4: 962–1023.

Evans, Gillian. 2016. *Educational failure and working class white children in Britain*. London: Palgrave Macmillan.

Fairchild, Amy L., and Eilen A. Tynan. 1994. "Policies of containment: Immigration in the era of AIDS." *American Journal of Public Health* 84, no. 12: 2011–2022.

Fairhead, James. 2014. "The significance of death, funerals and the after-life in Ebola-hit Sierra Leone, Guinea and Liberia: Anthropological insights into infection and social resistance." OpenDocs, October 10. https://opendocs.ids .ac.uk/opendocs/handle/123456789/4727.

———. 2016. "Understanding social resistance to the Ebola response in the forest region of the Republic of Guinea: An anthropological perspective." *African Studies Review* 59, no. 3: 7–31.

Faist, Thomas. 2008. "Migrants as transnational development agents: An inquiry into the newest round of the migration–development nexus." *Population, Space and Place* 14, no. 1: 21–42.

Farhi, Paul. 2014. "Media goes overtime on Ebola coverage but not necessarily overboard." *Washington Post*, October 6. https://www.washingtonpost.com /lifestyle/style/media-goes-overtime-on-ebola-coverage-but-not-necessarily -overboard/2014/10/06/d65e92fc-4d8a-11e4-8c24-487e92bc997b_story.html ?utm_term=.0606f8589bc8.

Farmer, Paul. 2014. "The largest ever epidemic of Ebola." *Reproductive Health Matters* 22, no. 44: 157–162.

Faul, Michelle. 2014. "The Village of Meliandou: Guinea's ground zero for the Ebola virus." *Vatican Radio*, December 10. http://www.archivioradiovaticana .va/storico/2014/12/10/the_village_of_meliandou_guineas_ground_zero_for _the_ebola_virus/en-1114310.

Feagin, Joe, and Zinobia Bennefield. 2014. "Systemic racism and US health care." *Social Science and Medicine* 103: 7–14.

Featherstone, David. 2013. "Black internationalism, subaltern cosmopolitanism, and the spatial politics of antifascism." *Annals of the Association of American Geographers* 103, no. 6: 1406–1420.

Fenner, Lukas, Rainer Weber, Robert Steffen, and Patricia Schlagenhauf. 2007. "Imported infectious disease and purpose of travel, Switzerland." *Emerging Infectious Diseases* 13, no. 2: 217–222.

Fidler, David P. 2001. "The globalization of public health: The first 100 years of international health diplomacy." *Bulletin of the World Health Organization* 79, no. 9: 842–849.

Fix, Michael, and Jeffery Passel. 1994. "Immigration and immigrants: Setting the record straight." *Urban Institute*, May 1. http://webarchive.urban.org /publications/305184.html.

Flynn, Gerard, and Susan Scutti. 2014. "Smuggled bushmeat is Ebola's backdoor to America." *Newsweek Global*, August 21. https://www.newsweek.com/2014/08/29/smuggled-bushmeat-ebolas-back-door-america-265668.html.

Fofana, Umaru. 2014. "Ebola center in Sierra Leone under guard after protest march." *Reuters*, July 26. http://www.reuters.com/article/us-health-ebola-africa-idUSKBN0FV0NL20140726.

Fox, Maggie. 2017. "Superspreaders drove Ebola epidemic, study finds." NBC News, February 13. http://www.nbcnews.com/storyline/ebola-virus-outbreak/superspreaders-drove-ebola-epidemic-study-finds-n720321.

Frost, Liz, and Paul Hoggett. 2008. "Human agency and social suffering." *Critical Social Policy* 28, no. 4: 438–460.

Fukuda-Parr, Sakiko. 2003. "The human development paradigm: Operationalizing Sen's ideas on capabilities." *Feminist Economics* 9, nos. 2–3: 301–317.

Fuller, Dawn. 2015. "How the Ebola scare stigmatized African immigrants in the US." *Medical Xpress*, November 2. http://medicalxpress.com/news/2015-11-ebola-stigmatized-african-immigrants.html.

Fuller, Jaime. 2014. "The Ebola travel ban is really politically popular. Here's why it's not happening." *Washington Post*, October 20. https://www.washingtonpost.com/news/the-fix/wp/2014/10/20/the-ebola-travel-ban-is-really-popular-heres-why-its-not-happening/?utm_term=.489e9bc8b279.

Gambino, Christine P., Edward N. Trevelyan, and John Thomas Fitzwater. 2014. "Foreign-born population from Africa, 2008–2012." US Department of Commerce, Economic and Statistics Administration, US Census Bureau. https://www2.census.gov/library/publications/2014/acs/acsbr12-16.pdf.

Gambino, Lauren. 2014a. "Airline cabin cleaners walk off jobs over Ebola fears at New York airport." *The Guardian*, October 9. https://www.theguardian.com/world/2014/oct/09/airline-cabin-cleaners-strike-over-ebola-fears-at-laguardia-airport.

———. 2014b. "Medical records reveal deceased Texas Ebola patient sent home with high fever." *The Guardian*, October 10. https://www.theguardian.com/world/2014/oct/10/thomas-duncan-ebola-medical-records-high-fever.

Gamson, William A. 1991. "Commitment and agency in social movements." *Sociological Forum* 6, no. 1: 27–50.

Garrett, Laurie. 2014. "Sierra Leone's Ebola epidemic is spiraling out of control." *Foreign Policy*, December 10. http://foreignpolicy.com/2014/12/10/sierra-leones-ebola-epidemic-is-spiraling-out-of-control/.

———. 2015. "Ebola's lessons: How the WHO mishandled the crisis." *Foreign Affairs*, September/October. https://www.foreignaffairs.com/articles/west-africa/2015-08-18/ebolas-lessons.

Garza, Lisa Maria, and Terry Wade. 2014. Ebola outbreak: Race to notify 131 other passengers on flight that carried second infected nurse. *Sydney Morning*

Herald, October 16. http://www.smh.com.au/world/ebola-outbreak-race-to
-notify-131-other-passengers-on-flight-that-carried-second-infected-nurse
-20141015-116pfb.html.

Gates, Bill. 2015. "The next epidemic—lessons from Ebola." *New England Journal of Medicine* 372, no. 15: 1381–1384.

Georges, Alain-Jean, Eric M. Leroy, André A. Renaut, Carol Tevi Benissan, René J. Nabias, Minh Trinh Ngoc, Paul I. Obiang, et al. 1999. "Ebola hemorrhagic fever outbreaks in Gabon, 1994–1997: Epidemiologic and health control issues." *Journal of Infectious Diseases* 179, Suppl. 1: S65-S75.

Gholipour, Bahar. 2014. "Ebola 'patient zero': How outbreak started from single child." *Live Science*, October 30. http://www.livescience.com/48527-ebola
-toddler-patient-zero.html.

Gire, Stephen K., Augustine Goba, Kristian G. Andersen, Rachel S. G. Sealfon, Daniel J. Park, Lansana Kanneh, Simbirie Jalloh, et al. 2014. "Genomic surveillance elucidates Ebola virus origin and transmission during the 2014 outbreak." *Science* 345, no. 6202: 1369–1372.

Goertzel, Ted. 2010. "Conspiracy theories in science: Conspiracy theories that target specific research can have serious consequences for public health and environmental policies." *EMBO reports* 11, no. 7: 493–499.

Goffman, Erving. 1963. *Stigma: Notes on the management of a spoiled identity.* London: Penguin Books.

Gomberg-Muñoz, Ruth. 2010. "Willing to work: Agency and vulnerability in an undocumented immigrant network." *American Anthropologist* 112, no. 2: 295–307.

Gong, Fang, Jun Xu, Kaori Fujishiro, and David T. Takeuchi. 2011. "A life course perspective on migration and mental health among Asian immigrants: The role of human agency." *Social Science and Medicine* 73, no. 11: 1618–1626.

Goodnough, Abby. 2014. "Countering fear of Ebola with education where West Africans live in the US," *New York Times*, October 2. https://www.nytimes
.com/2014/10/03/us/countering-fear-of-ebola-with-education-where-west
-africans-live-in-us.html.

Gordon, April. 1998. "The new diaspora—African immigration to the United States." *Journal of Global South Studies* 15, no. 1: 79–103.

Gordon, Milton M. 1961. "Assimilation in America: Theory and reality." *Daedalus* 90, no. 2: 263–285.

———. 1964. *Assimilation in American life.* New York: Oxford University Press, 1964.

Gornick, Marian E., Paul W. Eggers, Thomas W. Reilly, Renee M. Mentnech, Leslye K. Fitterman, Lawrence E. Kucken, and Bruce C. Vladeck. 1996. "Effects of race and income on mortality and use of services among Medicare beneficiaries." *New England Journal of Medicine* 335, no. 11: 791–799.

Gostin, Lawrence O., and Eric A. Friedman. 2015. "A retrospective and prospective analysis of the West African Ebola virus disease epidemic: Robust national health systems at the foundation and an empowered WHO at the apex." *Lancet* 385, no. 9980: 1902–1909.

Government Accountability Office (GAO). 2018. "Afghan and Iraqi special immigrants: More information on their resettlement outcomes would be beneficial." February. https://www.gao.gov/assets/700/690190.pdf.

Gozdziak, Elzbieta, Micah Bump, Julianne Duncan, Margaret MacDonnell, and Mindy B. Loiselle. 2006. "The trafficked child: Trauma and resilience." *Forced Migration Review* 25: 14–15.

Greeff, Abraham P., and Joanita Holtzkamp. 2007. "The prevalence of resilience in migrant families." *Family and Community Health* 30, no. 3: 189–200.

Greenman, Emily, and Yu Xie. 2008. "Is assimilation theory dead? The effect of assimilation on adolescent well-being." *Social Science Research* 37, no. 1: 109–137.

Greer, Scott L., and Phillip M. Singer. 2017. "The United States confronts Ebola: Suasion, executive action and fragmentation." *Health Economics, Policy and Law* 12, no. 1: 81–104.

Grey, Mark, and Michelle Devlin. 2015. "Ebola and localizing the 'global other' in the United States." *Somatosphere*, January 16. http://somatosphere.net/2015/01/ebola.html.

Guenther, Katja M., Sadie Pendaz, and Fortunata Songora Makene. 2011. "The impact of intersecting dimensions of inequality and identity on the racial status of Eastern African immigrants." *Sociological Forum* 26, no. 1: 98–120.

Guha, Ranajit, Gayatri Chakravorty Spivak, and Edward W. Said. 1988. *Selected subaltern studies*. New York: Oxford University Press.

Gushulak, Brian D., and Douglas W. MacPherson. 2004. "Globalization of infectious diseases: The impact of migration." *Clinical Infectious Diseases* 38, no. 12: 1742–1748.

———. 2006. "The basic principles of migration health: Population mobility and gaps in disease prevalence." *Emerging Themes in Epidemiology* 3, no. 3: 1–11.

Gussow, Zachary, and George S. Tracy. 1970. "Stigma and the leprosy phenomenon: The social history of a disease in the nineteenth and twentieth centuries." *Bulletin of the History of Medicine* 44, no. 5: 425–449.

Hadley, Craig, Ariel Zodhiates, and Daniel W. Sellen. 2007. "Acculturation, economics and food insecurity among refugees resettled in the USA: A case study of West African refugees." *Public Health Nutrition* 10, no. 4: 405–412.

Hagan, Elizabeth. 2014. "'My name is not Ebola': African children bullied at school." *New York Post*, October 27. https://nypost.com/2014/10/27/my-name-is-not-ebola-african-children-bullied-at-school/.

Haglage, Abby. 2014. "Kissing the corpses in Ebola country." *Daily Beast,* August 13. http://www.thedailybeast.com/kissing-the-corpses-in-ebola-country.

Hanna, Bill. 2014. "Possible Ebola contacts now up to 80." *Star-Telegram.* October 1. http://www.star-telegram.com/living/health-fitness/article 3875678.html.

Harris, D. R., Roxanne Andrews, and Anne Elixhauser. 1997. "Racial and gender differences in use of procedures for black and white hospitalized adults." *Ethnicity and Disease* 7, no. 2: 91–105.

Hays, Jo Nelson. 2009. *The burdens of disease: Epidemics and human response in western history.* New Brunswick, NJ: Rutgers University Press.

Healey, Joseph. 2010. *Race, ethnicity, gender, and class: The sociology of group conflict and change.* Thousand Oaks, CA: Pine Forge Press.

Hennessey-Fiske, Molly. 2014. "In Dallas, fear of Ebola seeps into daily routines." *Los Angeles Times,* October 16. http://www.latimes.com/nation/la-na-ebola -life-20141017-story.html.

Hersher, Rebecca. 2014. "Liberians wonder if Duncan's death was a result of racism." NPR, October 19. http://www.npr.org/sections/goatsandsoda/2014 /10/19/356986841/liberians-wonder-if-duncans-death-was-a-result-of-racism.

Herskovitz, Jon. 2014. "US parents confront fear of Ebola in classroom." *Reuters,* October 3. https://uk.reuters.com/article/us-health-ebola-usa-education/u-s -parents-confront-fear-of-ebola-in-classroom-idUKKCN0HS23C20141004.

Hewlett, Barry S., and Richard P. Amola. 2003. "Cultural contexts of Ebola in northern Uganda." *Emerging Infectious Diseases* 9, no. 10: 1242–1248.

Hoang, Lan Anh. 2011. "Gender identity and agency in migration decision- making: Evidence from Vietnam." *Journal of Ethnic and Migration Studies* 37, no. 9: 1441–1457.

Hollibaugh Jr., Gary E. 2017. "Presidential appointments and policy priorities." *Social Science Quarterly* 98, no. 1: 162–184.

Hopwood, Max, and Carla Treloar. 2008. "Resilient coping: Applying adaptive responses to prior adversity during treatment for hepatitis C infection." *Journal of Health Psychology* 13, no. 1: 17–27.

Hule, Jerome. 1999. "Africans protest killing of Guinean by New York Police." *All Africa,* February 10. http://allafrica.com/stories/199902100006.html.

Ibekwe, Nicholas. 2014a. "Ebola: Why Patrick Sawyer travelled to Nigeria— Wife." *Premium Times,* August 13. http://www.premiumtimesng.com/news /166660-ebola-why-patrick-sawyer-travelled-to-nigeria-wife.html.

———. 2014b. "Nigeria: Exclusive—How Liberian government cleared Patrick Sawyer to travel to Nigeria while under observation for Ebola." *All Africa,* August 12. http://allafrica.com/stories/201408120233.html.

Igonoh, Ada. 2015. "Flashback: How Sawyer passed Ebola on to Dr. Ada Ignonoh

and how she survived." *The Cable*, July 20. https://www.thecable.ng/how-i
-survived-ebola-2.

Iheduru, Adaobi C. 2013. "Examining the social distance between Africans and
African Americans: The role of internalized racism." PhD diss., Wright State
University.

International Organization for Migration (IOM). 2018. "IOM DR Congo Migration Health Division: Ebola response—North Kivu Situation Report 1."
International Organization for Migration, August 15. https://reliefweb.int/
report/democratic-republic-congo/iom-dr-congo-migration-health-division
-ebola-response-north-kivu.

Jacobson, Sherry. 1996. "TIGHT FIT—Families flood Vickery area, but former
singles' haven lacks services for children." *Dallas Morning News*, September
22, 1A.

———. 2006. "Neighborhood revival may hit roadblock." *Dallas Morning News*,
February 3, 1B.

———. 2014. "Ebola patient receives experimental treatment in Dallas hospital."
Dallas News, October 6. https://www.dallasnews.com/news/news/2014/10/06
/ebola-patient-receives-experimental-treatment-in-dallas-hospital.

Jimerson, Lorna. 2005. "Placism in NCLB—How rural children are left behind."
Equity and Excellence in Education 38, no. 3: 211–219.

Jin, Fang, Wei Wang, Liang Zhao, Edward R. Dougherty, Yang Cao, Chang-Tien
Lu, and Naren Ramakrishnan. 2014. "Misinformation propagation in the age
of Twitter." *IEEE Computer* 47, no. 12: 90–94.

Johnson, Rachel L., Somnath Saha, Jose J. Arbelaez, Mary Catherine Beach, and
Lisa A. Cooper. 2004. "Racial and ethnic differences in patient perceptions
of bias and cultural competence in health care." *Journal of General Internal
Medicine* 19, no. 2: 101–110.

Jones, Andrew Jerell. 2014. "Ebola fears turn into an epidemic of racism and
hysteria." *The Intercept*, October 21. https://theintercept.com/2014/10/21/cant
-ebola-become-latest-racist-national-security-issue/.

Jones, Esyllt W. 2005. " 'Co-operation in all human endeavour': Quarantine and
immigrant disease vectors in the 1918–1919 influenza pandemic in Winnipeg."
Canadian Bulletin of Medical History 22, no. 1: 57–82.

Jones, Kate E., Nikkita G. Patel, Marc A. Levy, Adam Storeygard, Deborah Balk,
John L. Gittleman, and Peter Daszak. 2008. "Global trends in emerging
infectious diseases." *Nature* 451, no. 7181: 990–993.

Jordan, Winthrop D. 2012. *White over black: American attitudes toward the Negro,
1550–1812*. Chapel Hill: University of North Carolina Press.

Joseph, Tiffany D. 2016. "What health care reform means for immigrants: Comparing the Affordable Care Act and Massachusetts health reforms." *Journal of
Health Politics, Policy and Law* 41, no. 1: 101–116.

Josephson, Erik, Yogesh Rajkotia, Eduardo Banzon, Andoh Adjei, and Francis Xavier. 2014. *National health insurance design in Liberia: Key considerations for equitable, efficient, and sustainable health care access.* November. Institute for Collaborative Development.

Käferstein, Fritz K., Y. Motarjemi, and D. W. Bettcher. 1997. "Foodborne disease control: A transnational challenge." *Emerging Infectious Diseases* 3, no. 4: 503–510.

Kalichman, Seth C. 2009. *Denying AIDS: Conspiracy theories, pseudoscience, and human tragedy.* New York: Springer.

Kang, Ezer, Bruce D. Rapkin, Robert H. Remien, Claude Ann Mellins, and Alina Oh. 2005. "Multiple dimensions of HIV stigma and psychological distress among Asians and Pacific Islanders living with HIV illness." *AIDS and Behavior* 9, no. 2: 145–154.

Katila, Saija, and Östen Wahlbeck. 2012. "The role of (transnational) social capital in the start-up processes of immigrant businesses: The case of Chinese and Turkish restaurant businesses in Finland." *International Small Business Journal* 30, no. 3: 294–309.

Keil, Roger, and Harris Ali. 2006. "Multiculturalism, racism and infectious disease in the global city: The experience of the 2003 SARS outbreak in Toronto." *Topia: Canadian Journal of Cultural Studies* 16: 23–49.

Kent, Mary Mederios. 2007. "Immigration and America's Black population." *Population Bulletin* 62, no. 4: 1–17.

Keohane, Robert O. 2002. "The globalization of informal violence, theories of world politics, and the 'liberalism of fear.'" *Dialogue IO* 1, no. 1: 29–43.

———. 2003. "Global governance and democratic accountability." https://www.researchgate.net/publication/228582436_Global_Governance_and_Democratic_Accountability.

Keusch, Gerald T., Joan Wilentz, and Arthur Kleinman. 2006. "Stigma and global health: Developing a research agenda." *Lancet* 367, no. 9509: 525–527.

Kim, Grace J., and Rev. Jesse Jackson. 2014. "Ebola outbreak and outcry: Saving Thomas Duncan." *Huffington Post,* October 7. http://www.huffingtonpost.com/grace-jisun-kim/ebola-outbreak-and-outcry_b_5943216.html?utm_hp_ref=tw.

Kim, Heejung S., David K. Sherman, and John A. Updegraff. 2016. "Fear of Ebola: The influence of collectivism on xenophobic threat responses." *Psychological Science* 27, no. 7: 935–944.

Kincaid, Cliff. 2014. "Ebola disinformation spread by leftist professor." *Accuracy in Academia,* October 28. https://www.academia.org/ebola-disinformation-spread-by-leftist-professor/.

Klabunde, Carrie N., Arnold L. Potosky, Linda C. Harlan, and Barnett S. Kramer. 1998. "Trends and black/white differences in treatment for nonmetastatic prostate cancer." *Medical Care* 36, no. 9: 1337–1348.

Koch, Tom. 2016. "Ebola in West Africa: Lessons we may have learned." *International Journal of Epidemiology* 45, no. 1: 5–12.

Kohn, George C. 2007. *Encyclopedia of plague and pestilence: From ancient times to the present*. 3rd ed. New York: Facts on File.

Kraut, Alan M. 2010. "Immigration, ethnicity, and the pandemic." *Public Health Reports* 125, Suppl. 3: 123–133.

Kreindler, Eric. 2010. "Thousands rally in Dallas for immigration reform." NBCDFW, May 3. http://www.nbcdfw.com/news/local/Thousands-Rally-in -Dallas-for-Immigration-Reform-92588199.html.

Kressin, Nancy R., Kristal L. Raymond, and Meredith Manze. 2008. "Perceptions of race/ethnicity-based discrimination: A review of measures and evaluation of their usefulness for the health care setting." *Journal of Health Care for the Poor and Underserved* 19, no. 3: 697–730.

Krieger, Nancy, Anna Kosheleva, Pamela D. Waterman, Jarvis T. Chen, and Karestan Koenen. 2011. "Racial discrimination, psychological distress, and self-rated health among US-born and foreign-born Black Americans." *American Journal of Public Health* 101, no. 9: 1704–1713.

Laccino, Ludovica. 2014. "Ebolaphobia: Guinean woman Fataomata Sompare attacked in Rome over virus fears." *International Business Times*, October 23. https://www.ibtimes.co.uk/ebolaphobia-guinean-woman-fataomata-sompare -attacked-rome-over-virus-fears-1471402.

Ladner, Jason T., Michael R. Wiley, Suzanne Mate, Gytis Dudas, Karla Prieto, Sean Lovett, Elyse R. Nagle, et al. 2015. "Evolution and spread of Ebola virus in Liberia, 2014–2015." *Cell Host and Microbe* 18, no. 6: 659–669.

Lambert, Bruce. 1990. "Now, no Haitians can donate blood." *New York Times*, March 14. http://www.nytimes.com/1990/03/14/us/now-no-haitians-can -donate-blood.html.

Landers, Jim. 2014. "Landers: CDC hopes Dallas cases will improve every hospital's practices." *Dallas News*, October 13. http://www.dallasnews.com /business/columnists/jim-landers/20141013-landers-cdc-hopes-dallas-cases -will-improve-every-hospitals-practices.ece.

Lau, J. T. F., X. Yang, H. Tsui, and J. H. Kim. 2003. "Monitoring community responses to the SARS epidemic in Hong Kong: From day 10 to day 62." *Journal of Epidemiology and Community Health* 57, no. 11: 864–870.

Lee-Kwan, Seung Hee, Nickolas DeLuca, Monica Adams, Matthew Dalling, Elizabeth Drevlow, Gladys Gassama, and Tina Davies. 2014. "Support services for survivors of Ebola virus disease—Sierra Leone, 2014." *Morbidity and Mortality Weekly Report* 63, no. 50: 1205–1206.

Leroy, Eric M., Alain Epelboin, Vital Mondonge, Xavier Pourrut, Jean-Paul Gonzalez, Jean-Jacques Muyembe-Tamfum, and Pierre Formenty. 2009. "Human Ebola outbreak resulting from direct exposure to fruit bats in Luebo,

Democratic Republic of Congo, 2007." *Vector-Borne and Zoonotic Diseases* 9, no. 6: 723–728.

Leung, Carrianne. 2008. "The yellow peril revisited: The impact of SARS on Chinese and Southeast Asian communities." *Resources for Feminist Research* 33, no. 1/2: 135–149.

Li, Y. H., and S. P. Chen. 2014. "Evolutionary history of Ebola virus." *Epidemiology and Infection* 142, no. 6: 1138–1145.

Lichter, Daniel T. 2013. "Integration or fragmentation? Racial diversity and the American future." *Demography* 50, no. 2: 359–391.

Link, Bruce G., and Jo C. Phelan. 2001. "Conceptualizing stigma." *Annual Review of Sociology* 27, no. 1: 363–385.

Littleton, Judith, Julie Park, and Linda Bryder. 2010. "The end of a plague? Tuberculosis in New Zealand." In *Plagues and epidemics: Infected spaces past and present*, edited by D. Ann Herring and Alan C. Swedlund, 119–136. Oxford: Berg.

Liu, Dandan, Ladson Hinton, Cindy Tran, Devon Hinton, and Judith C. Barker. 2008. "Reexamining the relationships among dementia, stigma, and aging in immigrant Chinese and Vietnamese family caregivers." *Journal of Cross-Cultural Gerontology* 23, no. 3: 283–299.

Lowe, Derk. 2014. "The deadly stupidities around Ebola." *Sciencemag* (blog). September 26. http://blogs.sciencemag.org/pipeline/archives/2014/09/26/the_deadly_stupidities_around_ebola.

Lowes, Robert. 2016. "CDC issues Zika travel alert." *Medscape*, January 15. https://www.medscape.com/viewarticle/857389.

Lozano, Rafael, Mohsen Naghavi, Kyle Foreman, Stephen Lim, Kenji Shibuya, Victor Aboyans, Jerry Abraham, et al. 2012. "Global and regional mortality from 235 causes of death for 20 age groups in 1990 and 2010: A systematic analysis for the Global Burden of Disease Study 2010." *Lancet* 380, no. 9859: 2095–2128.

Maes, Kenneth, and Ippolytos Kalofonos. 2013. "Becoming and remaining community health workers: Perspectives from Ethiopia and Mozambique." *Social Science and Medicine* 87: 52–59.

Maffly-Kipp, Laurie F. 2001. "An introduction to the church in the Southern Black community." *Documenting the American South*, May. http://docsouth.unc.edu/church/intro.html.

Majka, Lorraine, and Brendan Mullan. 2002. "Ethnic communities and ethnic organizations reconsidered: South-East Asians and Eastern Europeans in Chicago." *International Migration* 40, no. 2: 71–92.

Manguvo, Angellar, and Benford Mafuvadze. 2015. "The impact of traditional and religious practices on the spread of Ebola in West Africa: Time for a strategic shift." *Pan African Medical Journal* 22, Suppl. 1: 9.

Marc, Linda G., Alpa Patel-Larson, H. Irene Hall, Denise Hughes, Margarita Alegría, Georgette Jeanty, Yanick S. Eveillard, and Eustache Jean-Louis. 2010. "HIV among Haitian-born persons in the United States, 1985–2007." *AIDS* 24, no. 13: 2089–2097.

Maridor, Mathieu, Simon Ruch, Adrian Bangerter, and Véronique Emery. 2017. "Skepticism toward emerging infectious diseases and influenza vaccination intentions in nurses." *Journal of Health Communication* 22, no. 5: 386–394.

Markel, Howard. 1995. " 'Knocking out the Cholera': Cholera, class, and quarantines in New York City, 1892." *Bulletin of the History of Medicine* 69, no. 3: 420–457.

———. 1999. *Quarantine! East European Jewish Immigrants and the New York City Epidemics of 1892.* Baltimore: Johns Hopkins University Press.

———. 2009. *When germs travel: Six major epidemics that have invaded America and the fears they have unleashed.* New York: Vintage.

Markel, Howard, and Alexandra Minna Stern. 2002. "The foreignness of germs: The persistent association of immigrants and disease in American society." *Milbank Quarterly* 80, no. 4: 757–788.

Matthews, Stephen. 2018. "Ebola outbreak that has killed 75 in four weeks in the Democratic Republic of Congo has the potential to be the worst ever seen." *Daily Mail*, August 30. http://www.dailymail.co.uk/health/article-6114065 /Ebola-outbreak-DRC-potential-worst-seen.html.

Mayberry, Robert M., Fatima Mili, and Elizabeth Ofili. 2000. "Racial and ethnic differences in access to medical care." *Medical Care Research and Review* 57, Suppl. 1: 108–145.

McBrien, J. Lynn. 2005. "Educational needs and barriers for refugee students in the United States: A review of the literature." *Review of Educational Research* 75, no. 3: 329–364.

McCoy, Terrence. 2014. "A professor in the US is telling Liberians that the Defense Department 'manufactured' Ebola." *Washington Post*, September 26. https://www.washingtonpost.com/news/morning-mix/wp/2014/09/26/an -american-professor-is-telling-liberians-that-the-u-s-manufactured-ebola -outbreak/?utm_term=.b60512d0d1cb.

McGovern, Mike. 2014. "Bushmeat and the politics of disgust." *Cultural Anthropology*, October 7. https://legacy.culanth.org/fieldsights/588-bushmeat-and -the-politics-of-disgust.

McNeil, Donald. 2014. "Outbreak in Sierra Leone is tied to single funeral where 14 women were infected." *New York Times*, August 28. https://www.nytimes .com/2014/08/29/health/ebola-outbreak-in-sierra-leone-is-tied-to-one -funeral.html?_r=0.

———. 2016. "In reaction to Zika outbreak, echoes of polio." *New York Times*,

August, 29. https://www.nytimes.com/2016/08/30/health/zika-outbreak
-echoes-of-polio.html.

McNeill, William Hardy. 1998. *Plagues and peoples.* New York: Anchor Books.

Mercer, Claire, Ben Page, and Martin Evans, eds. 2013. *Development and the African diaspora: Place and the politics of home.* London: Zed Books.

Meyers, Jessica. 2008. "African refugees reshape Dallas' foreign population." *Dallas Morning News,* June 24. https://www.alipac.us/f19/african-refugees
-reshape-dallas-foreign-population-113668/.

Minkler, Meredith. 1999. "Personal responsibility for health? A review of the arguments and the evidence at century's end." *Health Education and Behavior* 26, no. 1: 121–141.

Molinet, Jason. 2014. "'Ebola!' High school soccer player from West Africa gets taunted during Pennsylvania game." *New York Daily News,* October 16. http://www.nydailynews.com/sports/high-school/ebola-high-school-soccer-player
-west-africa-taunted-pa-game-article-1.1976139.

Monson, Sarah. 2017. "Ebola as African: American media discourses of panic and otherization." *Africa Today* 63, no. 3: 3–27.

Moore, Ami R. 2013. *The American dream through the eyes of Black African immigrants in Texas.* Lanham, MD: University Press of America.

Moore, Thorn. 1991. "The African-American church: A source of empowerment, mutual help, and social change." *Prevention in Human Services* 10, no. 1: 147–167.

Morens, David M., and Anthony S. Fauci. 2013. "Emerging infectious diseases: Threats to human health and global stability." *PLoS Pathogens* 9, no. 7: e1003467.

Morens, David M., Gregory K. Folkers, and Anthony S. Fauci. 2004. "The challenge of emerging and re-emerging infectious diseases." *Nature* 430, no. 6996: 242–249.

Murdocca, Carmela. 2003. "When Ebola came to Canada: Race and the making of the respectable body." *Atlantis: Critical Studies in Gender, Culture and Social Justice* 27, no. 2: 24–31.

Myrdal, Gunnar, Richard Sterner, and Arnold Marshall Rose. 1964. *An American dilemma: The Negro in a White nation. The Negro social structure.* New York: McGraw-Hill.

Nelkin, Dorothy, and Sander L. Gilman. 1988. "Placing blame for devastating disease." *Social Research* 55, no. 3: 361–378.

Nelson, Steve. 2014. "Congressman: Close border to Ebola countries." *US News,* July 30. https://www.usnews.com/news/articles/2014/07/30/congressman
-close-border-to-ebola-countries.

Nolan, Markham, and Adi Cohen. 2014. "How a racist political hashtag spread

like the Ebola virus." *Vocativ.* October 14. http://www.vocativ.com/usa/us
-politics/obola-ebola-obama/.

Nurse, Earl, and Peter Guest. 2015. "How Sierra Leone plans to bounce back after
Ebola." CNN. December 23. http://www.cnn.com/2015/11/12/africa/sierra
-leone-ebola-recovery/.

Nuwayhid, Iman, Huda Zurayk, Rouham Yamout, and Chadi S. Cortas. 2011.
"Summer 2006 war on Lebanon: A lesson in community resilience." *Global
Public Health* 6, no. 5: 505–519.

Obermueller, Nele, and Angela Waters. 2014. "Ebola fears spark claims of racism
in Europe." *USA Today,* October 30. https://www.usatoday.com/story/news
/world/2014/10/30/berlin-immigrants-ebola-racism-africa/18187819/.

O'Carroll, Lisa. 2014. "Ebola epidemic: Sierra Leone quarantines a million
people." *The Guardian,* September 25. https://www.theguardian.com/world
/2014/sep/25/ebola-epidemic-sierra-leone-quarantine-un-united-nations.

Olausson, Ulrika. 2009. "Global warming—global responsibility? Media frames
of collective action and scientific certainty." *Public Understanding of Science*
18, no. 4: 421–436.

Omran, Abdel R. 2005. "The epidemiologic transition: A theory of the epidemiology of population change." *Milbank Quarterly* 83, no. 4: 731–757.

Onishi, Norimitsu, and Marc Santora. 2014. "Ebola patient in Dallas lied on
screening form, Liberians Airport official says." *New York Times,* October 2.
https://www.nytimes.com/2014/10/03/world/africa/dallas-ebola-patient
-thomas-duncan-airport-screening.html.

Opiniano, Jeremaiah M. 2005. "Filipinos doing diaspora philanthropy: The
development potential of transnational migration." *Asian and Pacific Migration Journal* 14, nos. 1–2: 225–241.

Pain, Rachel. 2009. "Globalized fear? Towards an emotional geopolitics." *Progress
in Human Geography* 33, no. 4: 466–486.

Palmer, Clare. 2011. "Place-historical narratives: Road—or roadblock—to sustain-
ability?" *Ethics, Policy and Environment* 14, no. 3: 345–359.

Panagiotakopulu, Eva. 2004. "Pharaonic Egypt and the origins of plague."
Journal of Biogeography 31, no. 2: 269–275.

Pappalardo, Joe. 2017. "5 surprising facts about immigrants in DFW." *Dallas
Observer,* February, 21. https://www.dallasobserver.com/news/5-surprising
-facts-about-immigrants-in-dfw-9206650.

Paradzai, Jealous. 2015. "A decolonial reading of the CNN framing of the Ebola
crisis." Midlands State University Institutional Repository. Master's thesis.
Midlands State University. http://ir.msu.ac.zw:8080/jspui/bitstream/11408
/2396/1/Paradzai.pdf.

Passewe, Sheila, Tonny Onyulo, and Jabeen Bhatti. 2014. "In Liberian slum,

Ebola quarantine magnifies misery." *USA Today*, November 2. http://www
.usatoday.com/story/news/world/2014/11/02/liberia-ebola-slum/18244091/.

Peddle, Nancy, C. Monteiro, V. Guluma, and T. E. A. Macaulay. 1999. "Trauma,
loss, and resilience in Africa: A psychosocial community based approach to
culturally sensitive healing." In *Honoring differences: Cultural issues in the
treatment of trauma and loss*, edited by K. Nader, N. Dubrow, and B. H.
Stamm, 121–149. Philadelphia: Brunner/Mazel.

Peters, B. Guy, and Brian W. Hogwood. 1985. "In search of the issue-attention
cycle." *Journal of Politics* 47, no. 1: 238–253.

Petersen, Eskild, Mary E. Wilson, Sok Touch, Brian McCloskey, Peter Mwaba,
Matthew Bates, Osman Dar, et al. 2016. "Rapid spread of Zika virus in the
Americas—Implications for public health preparedness for mass gatherings
at the 2016 Brazil Olympic Games." *International Journal of Infectious Diseases*
44: 11–15.

Petersen, Karen K. 2009. "Revisiting downs' issue-attention cycle: International
terrorism and US public opinion." *Journal of Strategic Security* 2, no. 4: 1–16.

PEW Forum. 2010. "Tolerance and tension: Islam and Christianity in sub-Saharan
Africa." Pew Research Center, April 15. http://www.pewforum.org/2010/04/15
/executive-summary-islam-and-christianity-in-sub-saharan-africa/.

Phelan, Jo C., Bruce G. Link, and John F. Dovidio. 2008. "Stigma and prejudice:
One animal or two?" *Social Science and Medicine* 67, no. 3: 358–367.

Phua, Kai-Lit, and Lai Kah Lee. 2005. "Meeting the challenge of epidemic
infectious disease outbreaks: An agenda for research." *Journal of Public Health
Policy* 26, no. 1: 122–132.

Picket, Steve. 2012. "Office shooting happened in high crime neighborhood."
CBS DFW, October 9. http://dfw.cbslocal.com/2012/10/09/officer-shooting
-happened-in-high-crime-neighborhood/.

Plautz, Jessica. 2014. "Air France crews petition to stop flights to Ebola-affected
countries." *Stuff News*, August 20. http://www.stuff.co.nz/travel/news
/60752913/Air-France-objects-to-flights-to-Ebola-hit-countries.

Plough, Alonzo, Jonathan E. Fielding, Anita Chandra, Malcolm Williams, David
Eisenman, Kenneth B. Wells, Grace Y. Law, Stella Fogleman, and Aizita
Magaña. 2013. "Building community disaster resilience: Perspectives from a
large urban county department of public health." *American Journal of Public
Health* 103, no. 7: 1190–1197.

Polesky, Andrea, and Gulshan Bhatia. 2003. "Ebola hemorrhagic fever in the era
of bioterrorism." *Seminars in Respiratory Infections* 18, no. 3: 206–215.

Poletto, Chiara, Marcelo F. C. Gomes, Ana Pastore y Piontti, Luca Rossi, Livio
Bioglio, Dennis L. Chao, Ira M. Longini, M. Elizabeth Halloran, Vittoria
Colizza, and Alessandro Vespignani. 2014. "Assessing the impact of travel

restrictions on international spread of the 2014 West African Ebola epidemic."
Euro Surveillance: European Communicable Disease Bulletin 19, no. 42: 1–6.

Portes, Alejandro. 1998. "Social capital: Its origins and applications in modern sociology." *Annual Review of Sociology* 24, no. 1: 1–24.

———. 2009. "Migration and development: Reconciling opposite views." *Ethnic and Racial Studies* 32, no. 1: 5–22.

Portes, Alejandro, and Leif Jensen. 1992. "Disproving the enclave hypothesis: Reply." *American Sociological Review* 57, no. 3: 418–420.

Portes, Alejandro, and Julia Sensenbrenner. 1993. "Embeddedness and immigration: Notes on the social determinants of economic action." *American Journal of Sociology* 98, no. 6: 1320–1350.

Portes, Alejandro, and Min Zhou. 1993. "The new second generation: Segmented assimilation and its variants." *Annals of the American Academy of Political and Social Science* 530, no. 1: 74–96.

Postell, William. 1951. *The health of slaves on southern plantations*. Baton Rouge: Louisiana State University Press.

Pourrut, Xavier, Brice Kumulungui, Tatiana Wittmann, Ghislain Moussavou, André Délicat, Philippe Yaba, Dieudonné Nkoghe, Jean-Paul Gonzalez, and Eric Maurice Leroy. 2005. "The natural history of Ebola virus in Africa." *Microbes and Infection* 7, nos. 7–8: 1005–1014.

Prakash, Gyan, 1994. "AHR Forum: Subaltern studies as postcolonial criticism." *American Historical Review* 99, no. 5: 1475–1490.

Preston, Richard. 1995. *The hot zone: A terrifying true story*. New York: Anchor.

Quist-Acton, Ofeibea. 2014. "Liberia lifts Ebola quarantine in Monrovia slum." NPR, September 3. http://www.npr.org/2014/09/03/345428525/liberian-authorities-try-ebola-awareness-campaigns.

Rabelo, Ionara, Virginia Lee, Mosoka P. Fallah, Moses Massaquoi, Iro Evlampidou, Rosa Crestani, Tom Decroo, Rafael Van den Bergh, and Nathalie Severy. 2016. "Psychological distress among Ebola survivors discharged from an Ebola treatment unit in Monrovia, Liberia—A qualitative study." *Frontiers in Public Health* 4: 142.

Ram, Ronki. 2004. "Untouchability in India with a difference: Ad Dharm, Dalit assertion, and caste conflicts in Punjab." *Asian Survey* 44, no. 6: 895–912.

Read, Jen'nan Ghazal, and Michael O. Emerson. 2005. "Racial context, black immigration and the US black/white health disparity." *Social Forces* 84, no. 1: 181–199.

Reed, Holly E., Catherine S. Andrzejewski, Nancy Luke, and Liza Fuentes. 2012. "The health of African immigrants in the US: Explaining the immigrant health advantage." Poster presented at the Annual Meeting of the Population Association of America, San Francisco.

Rees, David, Jill Murray, Gill Nelson, and Pam Sonnenberg. 2010. "Oscillating migration and the epidemics of silicosis, tuberculosis, and HIV infection in South African gold miners." *American Journal of Industrial Medicine* 53, no. 4: 398–404.

Reitmanova, Sylvia, and Diana L. Gustafson. 2008. " 'They can't understand it': Maternity health and care needs of immigrant Muslim women in St. John's, Newfoundland." *Maternal and Child Health Journal* 12, no. 1: 101–111.

Reuters. 2014a. "Ebola patient Thomas Eric Duncan vomited outdoors, witness tells Reuters." NBC News, June 25. https://www.nbcnews.com/storyline/ebola -virus-outbreak/ebola-patient-thomas-eric-duncan-vomited-outdoors -witness-tells-reuters-n216426.

———. 2014b. "Sierra Leone 'hero' doctor's death exposes slow Ebola response." Fox News. October 28. http://www.foxnews.com/health/2014/08/25/sierra -leone-hero-doctor-death-exposes-slow-ebola-response.html?refresh=true.

Richards, Paul. 2016. *Ebola: How a people's science helped end an epidemic.* Chicago: Zed Books.

Ridout, Travis N., Ashley C. Grosse, and Andrew M. Appleton. 2008. "News media use and Americans' perceptions of global threat." *British Journal of Political Science* 38, no. 4: 575–593.

Risse, Guenter. 1992. "A long pull, a strong pull, and all together: San Francisco and bubonic plague, 1907–1908." *Bulletin of the History of Medicine* 66, no. 2: 260–286.

———. 2017. "Grotesque appearances: 'The Chinese must go!' Perception of race and revulsion in San Francisco's Chinatown, 1849–1908." Unpublished lecture. https://www.researchgate.net/publication/312121818_Grotesque_Appearances _%27The_Chinese_Must_Go%27_Perception_of_Race_and_Revulsion_in _San_Francisco%27s_Chinatown_1849-1908.

Roos, Robert. 2014. "Migrations in West Africa seen as challenge to stopping Ebola." *Center for Infectious Disease Research and Policy,* November 14. http:// www.cidrap.umn.edu/news-perspective/2014/11/migrations-west-africa-seen -challenge-stopping-ebola.

Ross, Robert. 2014. *The borders of race in colonial South Africa.* New York: Cambridge University Press.

Rothkopf, Joanna. 2014. "Andrea Tantaros: Africans infected with Ebola might 'seek treatment from witch doctor.'" *Salon,* October 2. http://www.salon.com /2014/10/02/andrea_tantaros_africans_infected_with_ebola_might_seek _treatment_from_a_witch_doctor/.

Rouquet, Pierre, Jean-Marc Froment, Magdalena Bermejo, Annelisa Kilbourn, William Karesh, Patricia Reed, Brice Kumulungui, et al. 2005. "Wild animal mortality monitoring and human Ebola outbreaks, Gabon and Republic of Congo, 2001–2003." *Emerging Infectious Diseases* 11, no. 2: 283–290.

Rübsamen, Nicole, Stefanie Castell, Johannes Horn, André Karch, Jördis J. Ott,

Heike Raupach-Rosin, Beate Zoch, Gérard Krause, and Rafael T. Mikolajczyk. 2015. "Ebola risk perception in Germany, 2014." *Emerging Infectious Diseases* 21, no. 6: 1012–1018.

Ruger, Jennifer Prah. 2004. "Health and social justice." *Lancet* 364, no. 9439: 1075–1080.

———. 2007. "Rethinking equal access: Agency, quality, and norms." *Global Public Health* 2, no. 1 (2007): 78–96.

Ruggles, Steven, Katie Genadek, Ronald Goeken, Josiah Grover, and Matthew Sobek. 2017. "Integrated public use microdata series: Version 6.0 [dataset]. Minneapolis: University of Minnesota, 2015." https://usa.ipums.org/usa/.

Sach, Kevin. 2014. "Ebola victim's journey from Liberian War to fight for life in US." *New York Times*, October 5. https://www.nytimes.com/2014/10/06/us /ebola-victim-went-from-liberian-war-to-a-fight-for-life.html.

Sacramento, Igor, and Izamara Bastos Machado. 2015. "Immigration as a risk factor to health: Analysing Folha de S. Paulo's representation of an African immigrant during the Ebola outbreak." *Comunicação e Sociedade* 28: 49–71.

Sadeka, Sumaiya, Mohd Suhaimi Mohamad, Mohammad Imam Hasan Reza, Jamiah Manap, and Md Sujahangir Kabir Sarkar. 2015. "Social capital and disaster preparedness: Conceptual framework and linkage." *Social Science Research* 3: 38–48.

Salway, P., and W. Dell. 1955. "Plague at Athens." *Greece and Rome* 2, no. 2: 62–69.

Sanchez, Alonso, and Anne Marie Weiss-Armuch. 2003. "Study of North Texas immigrant communities." *Dallas International*, January 28. http://www .dfwinternational.org/resource_center/Study_of_North_Texas_Immigrant _Communities_2003.pdf.

Sargent, Greg. 2014. "Scott Brown: Anyone with Ebola can 'walk across' our 'porous' border." *Washington Post*, October 14. https://www.washingtonpost .com/blogs/plum-line/wp/2014/10/14/scott-brown-anyone-with-ebola-can -walk-across-our-porous-border/?utm_term=.999e7238f2fe.

Sartorius, Norman. 2002. "Iatrogenic stigma of mental illness: Begins with behaviour and attitudes of medical professionals, especially psychiatrists." *BMJ* 324: 1470–1471.

———. 2007. "Stigmatized illnesses and health care." *Croatian Medical Journal* 48, no. 3: 396–397.

Scheufele, Dietram A. 1999. "Framing as a theory of media effects." *Journal of Communication* 49, no. 1: 103–122.

Schmunis, G. A. 2007. "The globalization of Chagas disease." *ISBT Science Series* 2, no. 1: 6–11.

Schneider, Eric C., Alan M. Zaslavsky, and Arnold M. Epstein. 2002. "Racial disparities in the quality of care for enrollees in Medicare managed care." *Jama* 287, no. 10: 1288–1294.

Schrover, Marlou, and Floris Vermeulen. 2005. "Immigrant organisations." *Journal of Ethnic and Migration Studies* 31, no. 5: 823–832.

Selk, Avi. 2014. "Before his death, Duncan said he mistook Ebola case in Liberia for miscarriage; never lied." *Dallas Morning News*, October 8. https://www.dallasnews.com/news/news/2014/10/08/before-his-death-duncan-said-he-mistook-ebola-case-in-liberia-for-miscarriage-never-lied.

Sen, Amartya. 1999. *Development as freedom*. New York: Knopf.

Sernhede, Ove. 2014. "Youth rebellion and social mobilisation in Sweden." *Soundings* 56, no. 56: 81–91.

Sharma, Megha, Kapil Yadav, Nitika Yadav, and Keith C. Ferdinand. 2017. "Zika virus pandemic—Analysis of Facebook as a social media health information platform." *American Journal of Infection Control* 45, no. 3: 301–302.

Shavers, Vickie L., Pebbles Fagan, Dionne Jones, William M. P. Klein, Josephine Boyington, Carmen Moten, and Edward Rorie. 2012. "The state of research on racial/ethnic discrimination in the receipt of health care." *American Journal of Public Health* 102, no. 5: 953–966.

Shen, Yiqin. 2014. "'Little Liberia' market suffers on Staten Island." *Voices of New York*, September 26. https://voicesofny.org/2014/09/little-liberia-market-suffers-staten-island/.

Shuchman, Miriam. 2014. "Sierra Leone doctors call for better Ebola care for colleagues." *Lancet* 384, no. 9961: e67.

Singer, Audrey. 2015. "Metropolitan immigrant gateways revisited, 2014." Brookings, December 1. https://www.brookings.edu/research/metropolitan-immigrant-gateways-revisited-2014/.

Singh, Gopal K., and Barry A. Miller. 2004. "Health, life expectancy, and mortality patterns among immigrant populations in the United States." *Canadian Journal of Public Health* 95, no. 3: 14–21.

Siriwardhana, Chesmal, Shirwa Sheik Ali, Bayard Roberts, and Robert Stewart. 2014. "A systematic review of resilience and mental health outcomes of conflict-driven adult forced migrants." *Conflict and Health* 8, no. 1: 1–14.

Siu, Judy Yuen-man. 2008. "The SARS-associated stigma of SARS victims in the post-SARS era of Hong Kong." *Qualitative Health Research* 18, no. 6: 729–738.

Smith, Katherine F., Michael Goldberg, Samantha Rosenthal, Lynn Carlson, Jane Chen, Cici Chen, and Sohini Ramachandran. 2014. "Global rise in human infectious disease outbreaks." *Journal of the Royal Society Interface* 11, no. 101: 20140950.

Smith-Morris, Carolyn. 2017. "Epidemiological placism in public health emergencies: Ebola in two Dallas neighborhoods." *Social Science and Medicine* 179: 106–114.

Stafford, Mark C., and Richard R. Scott. 1986. "Stigma, deviance, and social control." In *The dilemma of difference*, edited by Stephen C. Ainlay, Gaylene Becker, and Lerita M. Coleman, 77–91. Boston: Springer.

Stein, Richard A. 2011. "Super-spreaders in infectious diseases." *International Journal of Infectious Diseases* 15, no. 8: e510-e513.

Sun, Lena, and Lenny Bernstein. 2018. "Ebola outbreak now at 105 cases, and bordering countries are on alert." *Washington Post*, August 14. https://www .washingtonpost.com/national/health-science/ebola-outbreak-now-at-105 -cases-and-bordering-countries-are-on-alert/2018/08/24/3b7a58a2-a7c2-11e8 -a656-943eefab5daf_story.html?utm_term=.c06ce77cce5b.

Swanson, Doug, Sarah Mervosh, Sherry Jacobson, Matthew Watkins, Tawnell Hobbs, Matthew Haag, and Robert Wilonsky. 2014. "Miscommunication at hospital led to Dallas Ebola patient's release." *Dallas News*, September 30. https://www.dallasnews.com/news/news/2014/09/30/miscommunication-at -hospital-led-to-dallas-ebola-patient-s-release.

Sy, Amadou, and Amy Copley. 2014. "The 2014 Ebola epidemic: Effects, response, and prospects for recovery." *Brown Journal of World Affairs* 21, no. 2: 199–214.

Takougang, Joseph, and Bassirou Tidjani. 2009. "Settlement patterns and organizations among African immigrants in the United States." *Journal of Global South Studies* 26, no. 1: 31–40.

Terkel, Amanda. 2014. "Hotline launches to help African immigrants facing Ebola stigma." *Huffington Post*, November 10. http://www.huffingtonpost .com/2014/11/10/ebola-stigma-hotline-african-communities-together_n _6133452.html.

Thiessen, Marc. 2014. "A 'Dark Winter' of Ebola terrorism?" *Washington Post*, October 20. https://www.washingtonpost.com/opinions/marc-thiessen -a-dark-winter-of-ebola-terrorism/2014/10/20/4ebfb1d8-5865-11e4-8264 -deed989ae9a2_story.html?utm_term=.c363b8083b4a.

Thompson, Andrew. 2001. "Nations, national identities and human agency: Putting people back into nations." *Sociological Review* 49, no. 1: 18–32.

Thompson, Nick, and Inez Torre. 2014. "Ebola virus: Countries with travel restrictions in place." CNN. November 4. http://www.cnn.com/2014/11/04 /world/ebola-virus-restrictions-map/.

Trauner, Joan B. 1978. "The Chinese as medical scapegoats in San Francisco, 1870–1905." *California History* 57, no. 1: 70–87.

Troh, Louise. 2015. *My spirit took you in: The romance that sparked an epidemic of fear*. New York: Weistein Books.

Tudor, Andrew. 2003. "A (macro) sociology of fear?" *Sociological Review* 51, no. 2: 238–256.

Tuttle, Brad. 2014. "8 ways somebody is making money off Ebola fears." *Money*, October 20. http://time.com/money/3525321/ebola-outbreak-products-fear/.

Ungar, Sheldon. 1998. "Hot crises and media reassurance: A comparison of emerging diseases and Ebola Zaire." *British Journal of Sociology* 49, no. 1: 36–56.

——. 2008. "Global bird flu communication: Hot crisis and media reassurance." *Science Communication* 29, no. 4: 472–497.

United Nations (UN). 1995. "Suspect cases of Ebola in Liberia." December 11. http://www.un.org/press/en/1995/19951211.h2888.html.

US Office of Refugee Resettlement. 2016. "FY 2015 served populations by state and country of origin (refugees only)." April 22. http://www.acf.hhs.gov /orr/resource/fy-2015-refugees-by-state-and-country-of-origin-all-served -populations.

Van Damme, Wim, and Wim Van Lerberghe. 2000. "Epidemics and fear." *Tropical Medicine and International Health* 5, no. 8: 511–514.

——. 2004. "Strengthening health services to control epidemics: Empirical evidence from Guinea on its cost-effectiveness." *Tropical Medicine and International Health* 9, no. 2: 281–291.

Van den Bulck, Jan, and Kathleen Custers. 2009. "Television exposure is related to fear of avian flu, an ecological study across 23 member states of the European Union." *European Journal of Public Health* 19, no. 4: 370–374.

Vang, Zoua M., and Irma T. Elo. 2013. "Exploring the health consequences of majority–minority neighborhoods: Minority diversity and birthweight among native-born and foreign-born blacks." *Social Science and Medicine* 97: 56–65.

Varia, Monali, Samantha Wilson, Shelly Sarwal, Allison McGeer, Effie Gournis, and Eleni Galanis. 2003. "Investigation of a nosocomial outbreak of severe acute respiratory syndrome (SARS) in Toronto, Canada." *Canadian Medical Association Journal* 169, no. 4: 285–292.

Venters, Homer, and Francesca Gany. 2011. "African immigrant health." *Journal of Immigrant and Minority Health* 13, no. 2: 333–344.

Wailoo, Keith. 2006. "Stigma, race, and disease in 20th century America." *Lancet* 367, no. 9509: 531–533.

Wallis, Patrick, and Brigitte Nerlich. 2005. "Disease metaphors in new epidemics: The UK media framing of the 2003 SARS epidemic." *Social Science and Medicine* 60, no. 11: 2629–2639.

Weeks, Joseph. 2014. "Exclusive: Ebola didn't have to kill Thomas Eric Duncan, nephew says." *Dallas News*, October. https://www.dallasnews.com/opinion /commentary/2014/10/14/exclusive-ebola-didnt-have-to-kill-thomas-eric -duncan-nephew-says.

Wei, Yingqi, and Vudayagiri N. Balasubramanyam. 2006. "Diaspora and development." *World Economy* 29, no. 11: 1599–1609.

Weiss, Jeffrey. 2014. "Confirmation of second Ebola case rattles Dallas." *Dallas*

News, October 12. http://www.dallasnews.com/news/metro/20141012
-confirmation-of-second-ebola-case-rattles-dallas.ece.

Wickramage, Kolitha, Sharika Peiris, and Suneth B. Agampodi. 2013. " 'Don't forget the migrants': Exploring preparedness and response strategies to combat the potential spread of MERS-CoV virus through migrant workers in Sri Lanka." *F1000Research* 2: 163.

Wilonsky, Robert. 2014. "Ebola patient's quarantined dog is hardly living the dog's life." *Dallas News*, October 14. http://www.dallasnews.com/news/metro/20141014-ebola-patients-quarantined-dog-is-hardly-living-the-dogs-life.ece.

Williams, David R., and Ronald Wyatt. 2015. "Racial bias in health care and health: Challenges and opportunities." *Jama* 314, no. 6: 555–556.

Williamson, Moira, and Lindsey Harrison. 2010. "Providing culturally appropriate care: A literature review." *International Journal of Nursing Studies* 47, no. 6: 761–769.

Witte, Kim, and Mike Allen. 2000. "A meta-analysis of fear appeals: Implications for effective public health campaigns." *Health Education and Behavior* 27, no. 5: 591–615.

Wong, Gary, Wenjun Liu, Yingxia Liu, Boping Zhou, Yuhai Bi, and George F. Gao. 2015. "MERS, SARS, and Ebola: The role of super-spreaders in infectious disease." *Cell Host and Microbe* 18, no. 4: 398–401.

World Health Organization (WHO). 1996. "Weekly epidemiological record." 71, no. 47: 353–360.

———. 2014a. "Ebola virus diseases update—Senegal." August 30. http://www.who.int/csr/don/2014_08_30_ebola/en/.

———. 2014b. "Mali case, Ebola imported from Guinea." November 10. http://www.who.int/mediacentre/news/ebola/10-november-2014-mali/en/.

———. 2015a. "Ebola in Sierra Leone: A slow start to an outbreak that eventually outpaced others." January. http://www.who.int/csr/disease/ebola/one-year-report/sierra-leone/en/.

———. 2015b. "Factors that contributed to the undetected spread of the Ebola virus and impeded rapid containment." January. http://www.who.int/csr/disease/ebola/one-year-report/factors/en/.

———. 2015c. "Origins of the 2014 Ebola epidemic." January. http://www.who.int/csr/disease/ebola/one-year-report/virus-origin/en/.

———. 2016a. "Ebola data and statistics—Situation summary on 11 May 2016." http://apps.who.int/gho/data/node.ebola-sitrep.ebola-summary?lang=en.

———. 2016b. "Ebola Situation Report—30 March 2016." http://apps.who.int/ebola/ebola-situation-reports.

———. 2017a. "Chikungunya—Italy." September 29. http://www.who.int/csr/don/29-september-2017-chikungunya-italy/en/.

———. 2017b. "Diphtheria-Cox's Bazar in Bangladesh." December 13. http://
www.who.int/csr/don/13-december-2017-diphtheria-bangladesh/en/.

———. 2017c. "Human infection with avian influenza A (H7N9) virus—China."
October 26. http://www.who.int/csr/don/26-october-2017-ah7n9-china/en/.

———. 2017d. "Middle East respiratory syndrome coronavirus (MERS-CoV)—
Saudi Arabia." December 19. http://www.who.int/csr/don/19-december-2017
-mers-saudi-arabia/en/.

———. 2018. "Cluster of presumptive Ebola cases in North Kivu in the Democratic Republic of the Congo." August 1. http://www.who.int/news-room
/detail/01-08-2018-cluster-of-presumptive-ebola-cases-in-north-kivu-in
-the-democratic-republic-of-the-congo.

World Health Organization Writing Group (WHOWG). 2006. "Non-pharma-
ceutical interventions for pandemic influenza, national and community
measures." *Emerging Infectious Diseases* 12, no. 1: 88–94.

Wyatt, H. V. 2011. "The 1916 New York City epidemic of poliomyelitis: Where did
the virus come from?" *Open Vaccine Journal* 4: 13–17.

Yin, Robert. 2013. *Case study research: Design and methods.* Thousand Oaks, CA:
Sage Publications.

Young, Michael. 2006. "Long-struggling Vickery Meadow showing promise—
Densely populated immigrant area getting aid with poverty, crime." *Dallas
Morning News*, January 8. 1A.

Zethraus, Lee. 1994. "Good neighbor policies—Martha Stowe helps Vickery
Meadow residents connect." *Dallas Morning News*, August 7. 21.

Zhou, Min. 1997. "Segmented assimilation: Issues, controversies, and recent
research on the new second generation." *International Migration Review* 31,
no. 4: 975–1008.

Zhou, Min, and Xi-Yuan Li. 2003. "Ethnic language schools and the development of supplementary education in the immigrant Chinese community in
the United States." *New Directions for Youth Development* 2003, no. 100:
57–73.

Zimmet, Paul. 2000. "Globalization, coca-colonization and the chronic disease
epidemic: Can the Doomsday scenario be averted?" *Journal of Internal
Medicine* 247, no. 3: 301–310.

Zirh, Besim Can. 2012. "Following the dead beyond the 'nation': A map for transnational Alevi funerary routes from Europe to Turkey." *Ethnic and Racial
Studies* 35, no. 10: 1758–1774.

Zong, Jie, and Jeanne Batalova. 2016. "Caribbean immigrants in the United
States." Migration Policy Institute. https://www.migrationpolicy.org/article
/caribbean-immigrants-united-states.

Index